Muscle head

By

William Brian Sved

Published by Terry Dog Books.

WELL-BEING:
THE STATE OF BEING COMFORTABLE, HEALTHY, OR HAPPY.

I dedicate this book to anyone who desires a more connected, enjoyable, and a healthier existence.

Acknowledgment

The title Muscle Head originates from when I was a teenager an expression my father used to say every time I would go to the gym and workout. He used to ask "Where are you going?" and every time I would reply to him, "To work out," to which he would reply, "You're going to be a Muscle Head.

Preface

I'd never thought much about writing a book, until approximately three years ago, the thought occurred to me. I have had so much of experience and adventure in my sixty-one years of existence. I have spent so much time and effort, exploring life's limits. Devoting my entire life to maintaining my inner spirit, I strongly desire to put all these thoughts on paper.

I am a free spirit. My soul is flushed with curiosity. I have a huge passion for living life to the limits and having moments that are filled with exuberance. I have lived my entire life with a deep discipline and passion for my own well-being. I thrive on being the healthiest, fittest me possible. I have overcome all adversities of life, committing to my own, and others' betterment.

My life has been an experiment on how far I could actually push myself, both physically and mentally. I have run marathons, competitively boxed, and rode motorcycles, all for the same reason. I wanted to feel alive. When you're pushing yourself through a marathon, facing your opponent in a boxing match, or riding a motorcycle, every cell in your entire body becomes alive and ultra-aware. I have experienced and enjoyed most forms of exercise to the fullest. I have maintained the same weight my entire life.

I started Personal Training in 1998. I trained all my clients with the same principles in mind to facilitates a sense of well-being in every one of them. Over many years of training my clients, my understanding of how to achieve the greater good has grown exponentially. I reached a point in my career where I created a formula that I happily applied to all my clients.

In the last several years, I have noticed that the common energy among people has changed. People have become affected by so many things. COVID-19 in 2020, higher prices, interest rate hikes, and the list goes on. Every time I would go on my computer, a message would pop up, asking for fast and quick solutions for people to feel better. It annoys me to no end, to witness the absolute nonsense and false information. Companies praying for cashing profits through the desperation of people.

That's why I decided to write this book. This is to represents the simple truth about what is really involved in any one, achieving a heightened sense of well- being. To understand that, every achievement must have a solid foundation behind it.

I wrote this book from my heart and from my deepest passion. I started writing two years ago. Writing for me, does not come easy. At times I really have to push myself and find that I am faced with the preverbal 'writer's block.' For me, it's like having constipation in the head. There is so much information percolating in my mind that it all gets backed up and nothing really comes out.

It happened to me after writing for a year and a half. I stopped writing and could not finish my book. I was actually resigned to the fact that it wouldn't be finished.

In February 2022, I went to visit my family who lived abroad. We were out for dinner one night and my Fifteen-year-old brother and I were talking about New York City, talking about the fact that he wanted to visit one day. I promised him that I would take him as I had been living in NYC for many years and could show him the city better than anyone.

We arranged a trip for mid-July, 2023. My brother arrived in Toronto on July 15, and on July 17, we loaded the car and off we went on his first road trip. NYC is about a nine-hour drive from Toronto. We, however, have a tradition of staying with my wife's sister who resides in Weston Connecticut which is one town over from Westport Conn, the quintessential New England town.

My sister-in-law, Vivian, owns an organic vegetable farm in Weston Conn. Many of the locals buy their fresh veggies from her. One of her customers and friends happens to be Mellisa Newman, Paul Newman's daughter, and her husband Raphael.

Upon planning our trip, I sent Vivian a message regarding our day of arrival and our plans to visit for a week. She sent me a reply that she was excited that we were finally coming after five years to visit her and her newly renovated beautiful home. When you stand in her backyard, you face a swamp that looks like you're in the Amazon jungle. She also asked if I would be interested in meeting Mellisa and Raphael. Well, Vivian knows what a huge, Paul Newman fan I am. When I was a very young child, my aunt took my sister and I to see Butch Casey and the Sundance Kid. A Western, starring Paul Newman and Robert Redford. It had a tremendous impact on me. I was star-struck. It was my first time seeing a movie in the theatre.

On our third day, we spent the entire day in Conn. In the mid-afternoon, I received a text from Raphael that he was at home and invited us to come over. I could not pass up this opportunity as Paul Newman has always been an icon to me. An actor I always admired and respected. I was very curious to see where he lived. I think I've watched ninety percent of all his movies. I was about a fifteen-minute drive away from his house, and both, my brother and I, hustled over to the original house that Paul Newman and his wife, Joanne Woodard lived in, for many years. We arrived to find a beautiful, charming, and old, England-style coach house, constructed on magnificent grounds. We both walked from the front driveway through an archway that has age-old ivy growing across, which leads to a pathway toward the front door.

I knocked once, and Raphael answered, welcoming me to his beautiful house. We were now, in Paul Newman's house, wow. Raphael, a very warm-hearted man, made us instantly comfortable with his warm greetings. As we entered the main part of the house, we could see pictures adorned on the walls, mostly of young Paul Newman and his wife, Joanne. The artistic energy in the house was alive and well. We had a short visit inside the house and then Raphael offered to walk us around. The property looked magnificent. There was a river that separated the two sides of the property and a suspension bridge, built to walk from one end to the other. The most important part of the grounds for me was the old tree house, built in a large tree in the middle of the backyard. There was a swinging bench that had many years of moss, growing on it.

The tree house was in the same condition. It was kept old, so to honor its authenticity. Raphael asked if I would like to go up the Treehouse and of course, I jumped over that opportunity. This is where Paul Newman spent his time, reading and relaxing. That was the main reason that he originally bought the house. We walked up the steps that led to an old wooden door with a pained glass window that almost felt like it would fall off at any moment, we entered the little room inside the tree house. Inside, was a charming old sofa, a lamp, a mirror, and that's it. It was so peaceful in that little room. The sun's glare glistened through the window that looked out onto the backside of the grounds. Here I am, sitting on the sofa that Paul Newman sat on, and the thought occurred to me that I needed to go home and finish my book. I thought to myself, if Paul Newman achieved so much and contributed to society in such a large way, why couldn't I finish writing my book. Why?

That's exactly what I did. It took me about another two months to complete. I needed a little inspiration. I am grateful to Raphael, who unknowingly inspired me! The truth is that finishing, doing anything in life, whether it's difficult or not, gives you a sense of accomplishment, a feeling of completion.

Contents

INTRODUCTION

In 1976, I was dispatched to an all-boys summer boarding school that was approximately a two-and-a-half-hour drive from my home. I was 14 years old. It was located in Northern Ontario, Canada, constructed on a beautiful body of water, named Lake Rosseau. A picture-perfect place. My Father, Mother, and baby sister chaperoned me on what was the longest drive of my 'so far short life.' The two-and-a-half-hour drive felt like a week. I was nervous. As we drove down the long, dirt-driven, and stony road that led to the school's entrance, I would always remember how fast my heart would beat and the thoughts in my head. I had never left my family, and especially my little sister, whom I was extremely protective of.

We walked around the grounds, which was pretty much what you would expect from a school in a small town in Northern Ontario. Log cabins, minimal luxury, that was it. It was a short walk to the lake. We were introduced to the faculty, my teachers, and the principal. Then, it was time to say goodbye. My heart raced fast. I was trying to hang on and stretch the inevitable fact that my family was leaving me here. I was so aware of every second that ticked along. I watched my family pull away from the drive out of the parking lot and back down the dirt road. Wow! What a weird feeling I remember having. I was faced with the reality that I was completely alone, fending for myself… well, absolutely for the first time. I could barely catch my breath! I felt like a helpless baby, left abandoned by its mother.

As I walked away from the parking lot toward the school, I could see other students at a distance. They were rough-looking kids who had seen a few fights, for sure. I noticed they were checking me out since I arrived, making facial gestures, and mocking me as I hugged my mother goodbye. I saw them pacing back and forth, as if stalking me. A person I had never seen before, walked up to me and spit right in my face. No one had ever spit in my face. Gobs of his saliva dripping down my face. I was appalled. I could not believe what he did. However, I knew that if I got into a fight in my first five minutes at School, it would be off to the Military Academy for

1

me. It took every ounce of self-respect and restraint I possessed to walk away from that, and I did. I was enraged. I was a pretty tough kid and didn't take crap from anyone. By the time I was twelve, I had already fractured my spine and broke my collar bone, which required a body cast for six months. My body had a major injury of some sort, that too, every six months. I promised my father that I would be a good boy, and I didn't want to disappoint him. It didn't take much time to figure out that this was no normal summer school. It was more like a juvenile detention center. It was a tough place with tough kids. A strict place with no tolerance for bad behaviors. All I could think about, was how I was going to get even with Mr. spitter. He humiliated me!

Next thing I did was go to the office and find out where I was bunking. One of the older students who was volunteering led me to my cabin. It was a large cabin with a small kitchen, two bedrooms, and a living room with a black and white T.V. My room was the last room down the hall and the smallest. Bunkbeds and a dresser, that's it. My roommate, who was lying on the bottom bed, had already arrived earlier in the day and had first dibs on the top or bottom bed. He chose the bottom, which meant I had to climb to the top. There was no ladder. He was there for the same reason I was, bad grades, delinquency, and a dislike for authority.

We immediately clicked. It seemed like we both spoke the same language. I was tired after chatting and meeting the other boys in the cabin. So, I thought I would get some rest, and as I was walking down the hallway toward my room, I passed the room next to mine. The door was open, the two older boys were staying in that room. They were lounging on the couch watching T.V. I peeked my head in the room, unaware that what I was about to see would have a lifelong impact on my entire being. In between two beds were a large poster thumb tac to the wall. It was a brilliant image of the late **great Bruce Lee**. The poster was from the movie, Enter the Dragon, where Bruce Lee was flexing his body in a fighting position with every muscle defined like that of a stealth leopard.

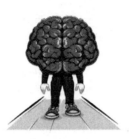

I was aware of Bruce Lee, I was a fan of the television show 'The Green Hornet,' in which Bruce Lee played Kato, the martial arts master, and the Green Hornets' side kick. I had never seen a poster of him before. I was absolutely mesmerized by this image of **strength** and **discipline** hanging on the wall before me. He was the fittest human I had ever seen. I couldn't believe that a person could be that powerful. I stared at that poster for at least 15 minutes before I was able to pull myself away, in fact, I went into that room every day of the summer term to see that poster. It inspired me. It spoke to me and expressed a belief that was already existing in my soul, a clear message of how I wanted to exist. I went back to my room and shuffled up to the top bed, where I lay wondering how many kids had been here before me, looking at the old wood ceiling. I wondered what they might have been thinking. How did they feel? Was I the only person who was afraid of being apart from their family. All I could think about was Mr. spitter and how I wanted to get back at him. I was getting angrier by the second, and that's when it occurred to me the light bulb went on sort speak. I was going to become like **Bruce Lee.**

I was going to be as fit, physically and mentally as he was. I thought that if I could to be as strong as he was that no one would ever spit in my face again ever. I really didn't know what to do with all these thoughts and emotions, it was over whelming. I remember thinking, perhaps, that I can make a promise to myself, If I made a promise to someone else, I would always keep it, I knew if I made a promise to myself, I would absolutely do my best to never break it. A promise always meant a great deal to me, even as a young boy, and it still does. I jumped out of bed and went into the bathroom, which was down the hall, locked the door, and stared into my eyes in the mirror. This was no ordinary moment. This wasn't just looking at yourself in the mirror.

When you really look deep into your own eyes, there's absolute honesty. It's like taking a dive into your own soul and swimming around a bit. I became very emotional, and I started crying, not a sad cry but a cry from feeling so connected to myself. After crying for a few minutes, a feeling of bliss overcame me, and that's when I made a promise to myself. I would always be as fit as possible, be ultra-aware, and always try to pursue strength of mind. Be as authentic, true, and connected to myself as I could. I would not let the world or anyone affect me. It is a promise that I have never broken to this day. That vision of Bruce Lee, his incredibly fit body, was chiseled into my brain forever.

That was the start of a deep, organic, and connected awareness of myself and my environment. I started doing pushups, jumping jacks, as well as running multiple times per day. Along with all the other activities that were amongst the school curriculum, Canoeing, swimming, etc., I was getting fit fast, and it felt **great!** I felt like Superman, and I couldn't wait till Mr. spitter picked on me again. This time, I was prepared. I wanted to try a different approach. I was doing very well at school, and I didn't want to blow it. I wanted to avoid having to fight this kid, so I decided that I was not going to allow him to provoke me. I would not give him the opportunity to get the better of me, I would keep my distance from him. During the second month of the summer term there was an annual run posted on the bulletin board in the lunch room.

There was a list of at least 25-30 students already signed up, and Mr. spitter was one of them. I thought to myself that this might be the opportunity to get back at him. He thought of himself to be the toughest kid around. If I 'whooped' his ass in a race, that might be my way of getting some retribution. I hadn't seen him much; he was a grade ahead of me and bunked in a cabin on the other side of the grounds. Non the less, whenever he saw me, he would make faces, hand gestures, and just act like a moron. I acted like he didn't exist. I could see it was driving him crazy that he

4

couldn't get a reaction from me. Race day arrived, and I awoke that morning very eager to put my new found strengths and beliefs into action.

This race was very important to me. I couldn't eat, I was way too anxious so I did a little bit of a warm up. I walked around the grounds a few times, then proceeded to the starting line, a chalk line applied by the gym teacher, a kind man who took his annual race very seriously. We were all instructed to place are left foot on the starting line and wait for his signal. I waited, completely focused on his command. **On your mark, get set, go!** I was like a hungry lion with its eye on a yummy gazelle. This was my opportunity, my moment. I started running as fast as I could, I was already a fast runner, but with Bruce Lee in my head, I was unstoppable. I ran so fast that when I turned around at the finish line, there wasn't anyone behind me, not for a long shot. I had come in first place and broke the time record for the course. It wasn't about winning the race for me it was more about my commitment to my promise. It was confirmation that I was on the right track. Winning the race meant that I was the fastest kid and probably by far the fittest. This empowered me to become the fittest me, possible. Summer term came to an end quicker than I expected. I ended up doing quite well academically that summer, and it taught me life lessons that I am forever grateful for. One of the most surprising lessons I learned was that I realized I was very capable of taking care of myself.

When I returned home, I became a Bruce Lee fanatic. There was no internet then, so any information about Bruce Lee was difficult to find. However, I managed to find some magazine articles and books about him, enough to have given me a sense of who exactly Bruce Lee was. I even used my mother's wooden broom stick to make my first pair of self-made nun chucks. I started running every day. I ran so for that my mother would follow me in her car, she was afraid I wouldn't find my way home or something. My interest in running lead to several marathons. Running a marathon is the closest you can get to your mind and body working in tandem. When your body gives up, your brain pushes you to the finish line, and vice versa. I have experienced both.

In 1997, I ran the New York Marathon and had a great run, finishing in good time. In 1999, I also ran the NYC marathon, and it was a completely different experience. It was a cold rainy day, the kind of rain that hits you right in the face when you are moving forward. When I reached the 22-mile point of the run, I hit the wall emotionally. Which means that your body has run out of fuel, and now your brain is telling you to stop. I ran the next 4 miles (a marathon is 26.2 miles), crying like a baby. I could not stop crying in fact, I almost crawled across the finish line. Spectators were offering me help. My strong will and discipline were what fueled me to the end. I also started playing tennis with my family at a club we joined, lots of tennis. In fact, my older brother was one of the top ranked provincial players in the province of Ontario. We spent the entire summer playing Tennis. It was a great alternative to sleep over summer camp, which didn't appeal to me or my siblings. Then I decided with my older brother and a friend to try Kung Fu. We joined a club in a unit of a warehousing complex called Twin Dragons. It was owned by two twins brothers who were Kung Fu masters, Mick and Martin McNamara. Our first-class Mick lined all the students up in a Straight line and told us to flex our Abdominal muscles as he proceeded to punch us all in the stomach as hard as he could. A few students threw up. That school taught me a lot about the discipline involved in martial arts. At 16, my sister and I started working out with weights at the tennis club, that had a separate sophisticated weight room for the era. That promise I made myself, manifested into having a life with great adventure and experimentation in how far I could push my body to do what my mind wanted, and my mind was able to drive my body.

By the time I was 22, I was married and had a baby on the way. I was an actor for some time, I performed in T.V. shows, theatre productions, a few movies, and many television commercials. My wife and I owned our own business, a high-end children's clothing store named Sassi Kids. I loved going on buying trips for the store. My wife and I went on a buying trip to the Gift Show in New York. It's a giant trade show. We were walking down one of the never-ending isles and noticed a T.V. monitor on a table playing a children's show about a purple dinosaur. We introduced our selves to the two Woman that were in the booth and ended up buying some of the videos for the store. We had known idea what that video tape would turn into. Approximately a month after returning from the trade show, the videos arrived. We put them out for sale and told our customers about them. The forty-eight videos that we had ordered were sold out within two weeks. We of course, immediately ordered many more. We had people driving several hours to our little store just for the Barney video. It was becoming a Craze. We went through so many videos that we became the distributors of Barney the dinosaur products in Canada when it was at its peak in popularity. I also became involved in the toy licensing business for many years.

In my mid-thirties, I was looking for another career, I felt it was time for change and I really had known idea what I wanted to do, and that's when fate came my way. I was having lunch with a friend after just having a workout together. Suzanne, was an actress friend from the industry, and we were also members of the same fitness club. We started chatting, and I mentioned how I wanted to find something that I could do that I had a passion toward. The same kind of passion I had for acting. She knew me quite well and very wisely suggested Personal Training. At that time, there were very few personal trainers, it was an industry that was in its infancy. Her suggestion made perfect sense to me, the only other thing that I had as much passion for as I did toward acting was fitness and my own well-being. I immediately signed up for an exercise physiology course at a local college. The course was 6 months long and had 4 day a week and one night schedule.

After the course had ended, I was determined to get a job at the best gym in the city which at the time was Bally's Total Fitness on Bloor St, which is the 5th Ave of Toronto. I was so determined to work there; I would not accept anything less. I was interviewed twice and had to wait a couple of months, but I was finally hired. After 6 months, I was the # 1 trainer in that particular location. I took my job very seriously, and before long, I had a waiting list of clients. I Was training 14 hours a day for many years. I became one of the top trainers in the whole company. After about 4 years, it was time for me to try and build a cliental outside of the gym. I wanted to have my own business and control my own destiny. I had already trained over 100 people, each person with unique situations and profiles.

I wanted to use my skills and knowledge to help as many clients as possible. It took me about three months to build a client base that allowed me to work 8 hours a day. I became one of the most sought-after Trainers in Toronto. I trained Top Models, Famous Actors, Hollywood Producers, CEOs of large corporations, and countless others. I will always push my boundaries and the obstacles before me. I have experienced great adventure and have pushed myself physically and mentally to a point where I have never felt more alive. One such adventure turned out to be a near death experience on a hiking trip on the John Muir trail. I was evacuated via helicopter and my life was saved by incredible doctors in Fresno, California. I will expand on this story further in the last chapters of the book.

Become the **best you** possible, and live your life with a **sense of well-being**, possessing more **energy** and a **higher life force.** I will present simple, logical solutions for reconnecting with your biological existence and a heightened feeling of being **alive! There** is no larger **reward** in life than maintaining **good health**.

Most information available today regarding **health** and **well-being** via the media and internet are either, outright scams or quick fix solutions for complex, deep, habitual-rooted issues. There is no such thing as a quick fix when it comes to a commitment for long-term change toward a more connected to self-lifestyle. Stop setting yourself up for failure with false expectations and misinformation.

You might have picked up this book amongst many others because you have a **desire** for change, and desire more **energy**. Perhaps you might want to lose body Fat and gain muscle mass or you just want to be more aware and enjoy life. Become more connected to your **biological self. You have in your hand's simple logical solutions toward changing your life. Tools to help navigate your journey to well-being.** Although it has become effortless and more immediate to do most things in our modern world, with the speed of technology out pacing **everything, it is increasingly more difficult to stay healthy both physically and mentally**.

In the United States, the Obesity rate from 2000-2018 rose from 30.5% to 42.4% for both male and female. At that same time, the prevalence of severe obesity increased from 4.7% to 9.2%. Obesity is responsible for health-related issues such as heart disease, diabetes high blood pressure, and mental illness. Why is there such a large part of our population that have lost touch with their own biological existence? Mental health issues are impairing a greater percentage of our population. Humans have advanced technologically at such a rapid pace that it has caused a shift in the common conscience. We expect things to be immediate. We have become **disconnected** from our responsibility to ourselves and our environment. Around every corner is temptation, **misinformation.** In fact, there is so much **misinformation** available at your fingertips that it causes confusion and mis trust.

There is an enormous amount of **temptation** on all levels and for every **desire.** In my experience as a Notable Top Personal Trainer to several hundred different clients **with** twenty-five years of **experience. I find myself at a point where my knowledge and instinct,** both physically and introspectively, **is** so finely honed that I could help anyone who **is** committed to finding a solution toward a sense of well-being. **I have been told that my energy is contagious, and am very enthusiastic in my profession. I have applied my awareness and knowledge** in altering the lives of many of my clients. **I instruct the same way I lead my life; I am a role model for others, and, therefore, can achieve a great deal of success.** Some simple choices and solutions can lead you to a more connected physical and mental reality. This book will discuss how anyone can achieve a more advanced sense of well-being. I will discuss how habit and discipline are the foundations for all solutions.

I

DESIRE AND BELIEF

Desire is "a strong feeling of wanting to have something or wishing for something to happen." A conscious impulse stimulated by or ignited via a thought, a visual picture. A stimulant of some sort. It is instinctual to have impulsive thoughts about your body's condition. It's your mind taking inventory of itself. The human body performs well when it is maintained well.

How does the desire for well-being manifest? Where does it come from? Are you thinking about an apparent change or motivated to make changes? Do you have a nagging, persistent thought or vision? What brings you to this point? It's **probably from a deep-rooted, emotionally attached desire to alter and improve** your well-being. It's natural to feel that way. There are many ways to manifest thoughts into reality. One of the best ones, in my experience, is actually to make a Plan, a contract with yourself. Write a promise to yourself, a commitment you genuinely believe in and are prepared to Honor. Put your thoughts on paper so that it's out of your head. Include in your contract what your intentions are and details of your desires. Date the contract and sign it. **Jim Carey,** the famous and multi-talented actor/comedian, told a great story about his commitment to himself. At the start of his career, he wrote a cheque to himself for Ten Million dollars. He carried it in his wallet for many years. Jim Carey was aware of his desire while writing the cheque. It was a way for him to recognize and facilitate his dream. His **passion** and **belief** in himself were so strong that it manifested into an unimaginable achievement.

Belief is "An acceptance that something exists or is true, especially without proof." There are many types of beliefs. For example, there is a collective belief where everyone believes the same thing. Religion and Money are examples. Then, everyone has their belief system. They think it to be true when it might not be the truth. Humans are very good at believing things because it satisfies their desires. Well-being is determined by how a person's desires are satisfied. Passion and belief must be integrated for an action to occur. If you genuinely believe that something can happen and desire to do it, anything is possible. Sometimes, our belief gets in the way of our desires, and strong desires can influence our beliefs.

Several years ago, I was on a climbing trip with my best friend, Mark, and his son, Luke. We were at a national park in Nevada called Red Rock Canyon. It's a 26-mile loop through very mountainous Terrain. We were there for several days as an annual mountain climbing festival was happening. There was a mix of novice and very serious climbers there. We were just beginners at best. On one of the days, we were in a group of 10 novice climbers being instructed on how to climb a 700-foot cliff straight up. We were taught everything from proper harnessing to anchoring, etc. Then, the instructor, a seasoned climber whose hands were like primate hands from all his years climbing, asked for a volunteer. I raised my hand the quickest and was selected. I had never climbed anything that high or level of difficulty before. I was naturally nervous. Here I am, helmet on, clamped in, and now I am looking straight up, and it's very high. At that moment, I told myself I could do this and started up this cliff. Every place I grabbed hold with my hands and feet was an affirmation that I was on my way up. My fear turned into courage, and I was at the top before I knew it. I think that people are conditioned to underestimate their capabilities. The reason I raised my hand the quickest was because I was afraid of the thought of climbing so high. I didn't want to give myself the opportunity for my fear to inhibit my desire.

Integrated Desire and Belief Equals Action.

Strength in your belief is based on the following:

1. Positive support.
2. Not having self-doubts.
3. More effort toward beliefs. The greater the belief, the greater the effort.
4. Education. The information helps motivation.

5. Persuasion from another source.
6. Belief in your ability is based on prior history. If you fail at something, it will likely affect your motivation.

I desired to overcome my fear, and I believed I could have the courage to achieve it. Unfortunately, our society's belief systems have become based on maybe even instant pleasure. Smoking cigarettes is terrible, but the desire is so vital for most people that they ignore the truth that it is a leading cause of death worldwide. A smoker's belief needs to change for their desire to be acted on.

Like the old saying, "It's easier said than done," turn the phrase around, "It's done, and now it's easier!"

There are five stages of change:

1. Pre-contemplation.
2. Contemplation.
3. Preparation for action.
4. Action.
5. Maintenance.

In my particular circumstance, at summer school, I desired to strengthen my body and mind. I believed I could empower myself to the same degree **Bruce Lee** had. It wasn't the picture of Bruce Lee that motivated me. It was what the image represented to me. I knew that my mind would follow if I made my physical being more strengthened.

We all know how to fulfill a desire. The problem is that we are conditioned to prioritize the wrong wants, most being pleasure-orientated. Marketing and the media have a great deal of influence on our desires. Humans have a tremendous appetite for acquiring stuff/possessions. Nike is an excellent example of a company that beautifully markets their products. They use the best athletes in the world to promote their products. Nike products are advertised to appeal to a consumer's desire for physical betterment. When you go into a sporting goods store to purchase a pair of Nike shoes, most people already know the shoe they desire. They do not need a salesperson to sell them sneakers but provide the customer with what they need. The opposite example is a person who goes into a sports store without knowing what shoe they want. They rely on the salesperson to provide them with what they desire. They need to be educated on what they need.

A tremendous amount of advertising and marketing is geared toward well-being. Companies influence your desire by using false advertising information and sexy models with perfect bodies. "Get a six-pack in 30 days" and "Lose 50 pounds in 30 days" are just a few examples. As I discussed earlier, there is no such thing as a quick-fix solution to your self-betterment. Avoid advertising that offers quick fixes. Be careful and stay clear of what I refer to as set-up words. Words that have expectations hidden within their meaning. **Diet** is one of them. You're sadly mistaken if you think diet alone will be the answer to a well-rounded, realistic approach. I wouldn't say I like to use the word diet. It creates false expectations. Diet means "the kind of food that a person, animal, or community habitually eats." Sustenance is a complex and complicated matter that will be discussed in further detail in other chapters.

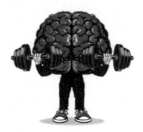

By definition, for the desire to be realized, something has to be done. Some action needs to occur. Nothing happens without action or movement.

The average human has many thousands of thoughts per day. Most of those thoughts could be better spent on something other than insignificant information, perhaps even negative reviews. It's best to change negative thoughts into positive, self-promoting thoughts. Start researching information that relates to your desire. Increase your knowledge and thus increase the number of studies related to your betterment. Now, you are on the right path. The more you start thinking and researching any desire, the more likely you are to act on your thoughts. Achievement of any nature occurs when readiness meets opportunity. Start thinking about your passion. Start making opportunities! Connect with people that will have a positive effect and encourage your progression. Socialize in environments that are helpful in your pursuit of well-being, join a fitness club, go to health food stores, and buy yourself a new pair of sneakers.

Keep things simple. Don't complicate your journey with unrealistic goals. I interviewed with a 35-year-old female many years ago. I asked her what her plans were. She handed me a picture of a famous top model in a bathing suit with a perfect body. At first, I thought she was joking, but she was dead serious. This woman was 50 pounds overweight and had never exercised a day. I told her that her expectation was unrealistic and that she was setting herself up for disappointment. I advised her to create a more organic and realistic vision of herself. To be the best she could be. After a long conversation, we agreed to work together, and a few days later, I structured a plan for her in the form of a contract, and she accepted. I trained her for many years, and to this day, she remains determined to continue working on her well-being. I recommend slowly working your way up the never-ending pyramid to well-being. The best and most effective way to start something is to attack it on every level, a little at a time. Start exercising and, at the same time, work on your nutrition, stress levels, sleeping habits, and water intake.

The average human body is made up of 30,000,000,000,000 trillion cells that work well in harmony and are responsible for carrying out all the necessary functions to sustain life. There are several hundred different types of cells. Fat, skin, and brain cells are just a few examples. Brain cells are, in fact, more prominent to send signals quickly. All cells are specialized to perform unique functions. Humans are very complex creatures that require regular maintenance. Like anything else, the more you maintain it, the longer it lasts. Exercise, Proper eating habits, and stress management lead to healthier cells and healthier cells, meaning an **improved** and a **healthier** you!

II

BEHAVIORAL CHANGE, HABIT FORMING AND

DISCIPLINE

Behavior is defined as "The way in which one acts or conducts oneself." From early on in our infancy and until the moment we die, our behavior constantly evolves. For the most part, our behavior might be completely different from year to year or even from day to day. Behavior is determined through many different components. Self-evaluation is essential. Have you ever evaluated yourself toward healthy behavior for both, your mind and body? Environment is "The surroundings or conditions in which a person, animal or plant, lives or operates." Hence, your environment directly effects your behavior.

Your ability for behavioral change is based on the following:

1. **Time:** Do you have the time to initiate the behavior? If not, then make time!
2. **Resource:** Do you have the financial ability to initiate behavior? If not financial, then what other resources do you rely on?
3. **Physical Effort:** Do you have the time to bring physical effort to help change your behavior?
4. **Education:** Sufficient information on behavioral change promotes positive growth of the mind and body.
5. **Planned Behavioral Change:** Make a plan toward healthier environmental choices. To greater extents, your ability is based on prior successes and/or failures, and the current **state of mind**. It is also essential to stay away from negative information and negative judgement from others. The attitudes and social pressures also influence the shape of your intentions and impulse.

Routine, "The Sequence of actions regularly followed."

Behavior has to be regularly analyzed in order for it to become a habit. A routine is something that takes effort. One of the most effective ways to stimulate behavioral change is to alter the routine. Routine refers to the chain of events that dictates behavior. If you don't want to drink alcohol, don't go to a bar. If you don't want to eat junk food, don't go to a fast food restaurant. Develop reminders or alarms to initiate change. In order to take action and change behavior, I used to instruct my clients to post notes all over the house, precisely, everywhere. With cell phones, you can easily set all sorts of reminders to do things. Visual triggers are highly effective. It is best to try, envision the behavior you would like to acquire. Triggers are very effective when you're faced with temptation toward unwanted behaviors. Therefore, behavior has to be regularly executed in order to form habit.

Behavioral picky back helps you choose a daily routine that you do every day and would like it to change. Let's say you're on your phone way too much and you want to devote more time to something that is essentially constructive. When you are on your phone, drink 8-ounce glass of water or walk while you talk. This what I call picky back behavior. Doing something that is routine and adding a positive routine attached to it.

The amount of effort expended toward a change in behavior is equal to its result. An example of this is if you choose to stop drinking Soda. A 100% effort would be to never drink another Soda again. A 50% effort would be to have less soda and, so on. The realistic approach lies somewhere in between. Most people find it very difficult to make a 100% change. In my experience, the most effective way for behavioral change is to take baby steps. I instructed my clients to make a realistic change and one that wasn't too difficult. With the Soda example, my approach was to cut back on the amount over time. For instance, instead of consuming two a day, have one every other day and slowly phase out the soda with a better, healthier choice. It takes less effort and creates less stress than to try and completely change a behavior. The more you believe in yourself, the chances for effort are far greater. Behavioral change requires repetition in order to form, and/or alter habits!

Habit, "A settled tendency or usual manner of behavior."

"A behavioral pattern acquired by frequent repetition. Habit forming is based on behavioral change. Habits are ingrained in our everyday lives and are performed with very little effort. You know it's a habit when you feel uncomfortable without it.

Positive behavioral change and positive habit-forming equals discipline

Habit	Replacement
Fast Food	Home-made food
Toxic people	Mentors positive people
Complaining	Gratitude or appreciation
Overthinking	Action
Blame	Responsibility
Negative Thoughts	Positive thoughts.

21 Day Habit Re-Set Plan

Use post-it notes for reminders. It's best to place them where you will notice them easily, such as on your wallet, refrigerator, bathroom mirror or on the back of your cell phone. This is how your post- it notes should look.

I WILL: This enunciates whatever it is that you want to do, when you're going to do it, if today, and what the reward is. For example, if you drink four cups of coffee per day, post a note on your phone.

Today, I will eliminate one cup of coffee and replace it with a glass of water, The reward is, you're adding a glass of water to your daily routine, which has positive effect on your well-being. Enlisted are some 'notes to self' that perform best if worked upon daily.

Days	Note To Self
Day 1	I will walk around the block for at least 10 Minutes, that equals 500 steps. I will drink one glass of water (8 oz) of water.

Day 2	I will wake up and appreciate the day. I will drink a glass of water. I will do one pushup, the pushups are referred to proper form, further described in Chapter 4, Exercise.
Day 3	I will walk around the block twice, drink a glass of water, get a good night sleep. 8 hours is sleep is optimal for a better functioning mind and body.
Day 4	I will do 2-3 pushups, three times during the day. I will drink a glass of water, and cook a meal. A healthy meal that includes healthy carbs, protein, and fat. From this day forward, you should be drinking at least a Litre of water Per day.
Day 5	I will walk around the block, three times today. I will drink one and a half glass of water, alter one unhealthy snack for another healthier choice. For instance, a piece of fruit instead of a candy.
Day 6	I will do one random act of kindness.
Day7	I will walk around the block three times, approximately 1500 steps.
Day 8	I will do 3 lunges for each leg, this section is referred to proper form explained in Chapter 3, and do 3 push-ups.
Day 9	I will walk around the block four times, eliminate one unhealthy food choice, and replace it with a healthier one.
Day 10	I will think about a healthy hobby and do some research on it.
Day 11	I will walk around the block 5 times, and do 5 push-ups.
Day 12	I will walk around the block 6 times, and do 5 wall squats.
Day 13	I will walk around the block 7 times, do 5 push-ups, 5 triceps, and Dips.
Day 14.	I will walk around the block 8 times.
Day 15	I will walk around the block 9 times, do 6 push-ups, 6 ball squats, and a 10 second plank.

Day 16.	I will walk around the block 10 times.
Day 17	I will walk around the block 10 times, do 7 push-ups, 7 ball squats and 20 second plank.
Day 18	I will walk around the block 11 times.
Day 19	I will walk around the block 12 times, do 8 push-ups, 8 ball squats, and a 20 second plank.
Day 20	I will walk for 30-40 mins nonstop, approximately making 10,000 steps.
Day 21	I will walk for 1 hour nonstop.

Congratulations. If you have followed this plan, you have disciplined yourself and have created a new routine which will eventually become a habit in the longer run.

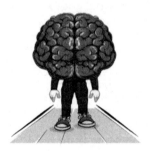

At the same time infants start forming habits, they also start the process of becoming aware of their environment and their awareness of space. This development is called **proprioception.** Proprioception is the body's ability to sense Movement, Action and location. It is present in every body movement you have. Without proprioception, you wouldn't be able to move without thinking about your next step. A good example would be if you lived in your environment, say maybe an apartment or house for a long period of time, and you know exactly where everything is placed around the house. Let's say you were to awaken in the middle of the night to use the lavatory, you could, most likely do it with the lights off and your eyes, closed. You are highly aware of the exact amount of space you're in. Location of the walls, toilet etc. You could also, most likely find your tooth brush and paste, brush your teeth, rinse your mouth and all in the dark with your eyes closed. If you have never done that, you should try it and see how closely you can relate to my example.

By the time you're an adult, your way of movement , your awareness of your space, and your location in that space are all based on your behavior and habit. You become highly aware, but only within the parameters of your own habits. What I mean by this is you probably Eat at the same time every day, shower ,dress and all the other pattern of habits within your day. These are habits that you could act on with minimal amount of thought and physical effort. If you make dinner in your own kitchen, and you know precisely where everything is, its gets easier to whip up a quick, good meal but if you were to cook in another unfamiliar kitchen, it would be much more complicated. Exercise and a pursuit of well-being of any kind promotes a heightened awareness of self and space.

Don't make any routine you want to develop, too difficult to initiate. If you have never walked and desire to start a walking routine. Start walking every day for 10 mins and over time progress to walking further. It's easier to form a habit if you make it easy on both, your body and mind. Sometimes you are forced to break habits due to health reasons and change of environment. However, the longer the habit exists, the harder it is to unload or alter. Habits that are pleasure based, are harder to change.

The average amount of time to form a habit varies for each person. Some habits are easy to form while others are quite hard. In my own experience, the amount of time to form habits was based on many things but the most important is **consistency, consistency, consistency!** The more consistent a client is, the greater the opportunity in forming and altering habits. If a client started strong for 1 month then for a number of reasons wasn't consistent, it adversely impacts the amount of time it took them to form a habit. If you disrupt the progression of a new habit, it's like taking a step backwards and losing your momentum. A good example of this is when you see a sports team that is on a winning streak, the team has so much energy, discipline, talent, and momentum behind them that in itself propels them forward. Gaining momentum, physically, and mentally keeps you on track, like a train roaring down the track, either get on or get outa the way. If you disrupt that momentum, perhaps a player or two gets injured or a couple of losses in a row, has an effect on the overall team as a whole.

Momentum, is the impetus gained buy a moving object. If you roll a ball down a hill, it gains momentum until it is stopped . When the ball is stopped, it regains its momentum every time it is stopped. Likewise, the same theory applies to humans forming habits.

Impetus: Something that makes a process or activity happen or happen more quickly.

Consistency is the Impetus of Well-being!

I myself have had a consistent commitment to my own well-being my entire life. In fact, since I was twelve years old. My own behavior is predicated on my deep-rooted habits. My habits serve me on a higher level and my commitment to my habits gives me a feeling of well-being. I try to make all my choices based on my belief. I became a vegetarian many years ago. I haven't eaten a piece of meat since. It gives me a feeling of well-being because I connect to my true belief and how I want to exist. My motivator is my understanding to not comply with my promise to myself would make me feel disappointed in Myself. My habits transformed into astounding discipline!!

Discipline: To train or develop by instruction and exercise especially in self-control. "Orderly, or prescribed conduct or pattern of behavior."

The most underrated aspect of any achievement is discipline. In my pursuit of becoming the most capable trainer, I devoted a lot of time, effort, and thought about what it was that was actually giving my clients a sense of well-being. It was obviously based to a great deal on visual. The actual visual change was something that they could see but more importantly what about the things they could not see. Firstly, the changes on a cellular level as well as the betterment of your whole inner being, the things you can't see. The things that people could see didn't satisfy them as much as the things they could feel both physically and mentally. That's where discipline comes in picture. Over the span of many years, I understood and communicated to every one of my clients that their improvements and in a lot of cases their transformed physical strength gave their mind a gift and that gift was discipline. Discipline gives you a feeling of accomplishment, a feeling that you are righteous for your commitment to your own betterment, gives you a feeling of honor. That's a powerful thing. You can always count on Discipline. Even when you're not emotionally motivated, it will never let you down. Discipline is the segway between desire and belief and behavior and habit! It is your default page and something you can always rely on. It is the bridge between Goals and Achievements.

Goal, The object of a person's ambition or effort, an aim or desired result, the destination of a journey.

Discipline, is responsible for any achievements humans have or will create. Buildings are built on the discipline and expertise of its creators. Companies are successful based on the discipline of its workers and Entrepreneurs. Athletes who are at the top of their game are there from sheer discipline. They have the talent but without extreme discipline they would not be able to compete on a world class level. My favorite athlete of all times, Bjorn Borg was the number one tennis player for many years. He actually had quite an unorthodox style. He was quite a talented Athlete. The characteristic that set him apart from all the other great tennis players at that time, mostly Late 1970's and early 80's. He was fitter than any other player on the circuit, all because of his habitual discipline. Practicing many hours, a day, every day. When he was young, apparently his pulse rate was measured to be 37 bpm at rest. He garnered the nickname the "**Iceman**" because of his discipline toward his focus. He showed no emotion during a match because he was so focused. I actually was fortunate enough to have met him at the major tournament held yearly in Toronto. I was 17 years old and my brother and I were drivers for the players. My brother was a top ranked tennis player in Canada. We escorted players to and from the airport and to their hotels. We also picked up a young, Jhon McEnroe at the airport coming in from New York. He was quite the character. First thing he did when he got into the car, I was in the back seat and my brother was driving, he whipped out a joint and started smoking it while he bad mouthed his Canadian opponent who he was en route to play against. He was a fantastic athlete and rose to be number one tennis player in the world as a result of discipline. According to theories, if you discipline yourself to practice or perform something for 10,000 hours that you would qualify to compete and perform at the highest levels of anything.

In the context of how discipline relates to well-being, discipline is the foundation, the roots of what is really the inherent reason for improvement on a physical and mental level. The same way that the tennis players applied their discipline into practice. They became mentally and physically strong, one bolsters the other. In other words, the more you practice or apply yourself, physically and mentally the more you evolve toward a **symbiotic balance of both**.

A handful of my clients were extremely wealthy, successful business men and woman. They all controlled very large companies. They all had one thing in common, they had so much responsibility to their work. They were so involved in their business that their minds were far more capable than their physical bodies. They were always under a high level of stress and mental involvement. Some were so involved they couldn't even leave the house for a power walk without their cell phones because they were always on call sort of speak. I was on a Power walk with one of these clients and he was constantly on his phone. It really bothered me. The next session we had, I explained to him that I did not want him bringing his phone because I found it counterproductive. I ended up insisting that he shouldn't have brought his phone, which he did with much resistance. It was for his betterment and I think he realized that. He was like a child without their teddy bear. One of my objectives was to get my clients out of their environment away from distractions. Your environment is actually more responsible in your ability to act on an impulse than you think. Are you a busy person with a schedule that allows for no free time or relaxation or freedom of thought. Do you have huge responsibilities. If you fit into this category and most people do, then your impulses are harder to act on, your environment is invading your desire, sort of speak. Altering your environment as much as possible is a very integral component in manifesting a desire.

I also wanted to utilize the time we had to talk with them and get them attached to thinking outside the parameters in which they behaved. He and all the other clients with that same profile couldn't do it. They could not walk without their phones. It was amazing to me. I was compelled to find out why. So, I started thinking maybe obsessing a little actually to figure out what was at the bottom of such commonalities. I did a lot of thinking and I came to a conclusion. These people had so much other responsibility to other things other than themselves that they prioritized everything over their physical being. Their bodies were suffering from lack of any activity or movement but also from so intensely using their brain. They all were highly intelligent people, However, they were virtually completely unaware of their physical well-being. They were completely unbalanced and on the road to disaster, in terms of their health. Surprisingly a large percentage were all what I call Yo Yo Clients. They were like a Yo Yo, they went up and down in their consistency. What intrigued me most was that these people were so highly motivated and disciplined in their work ethic but however, they did not have that same discipline toward their own well-being. I suppose there is only a certain amount of discipline a person can sustain. Discipline takes effort and humans have a limited amount of energy. In this particular case, their mental state drained their physical sate. The opposite scenario also occurs when you are too physical but aren't mentally stimulated enough. I guess it goes back to **Yin and Yang every positive side has a negative side**. It's what make us human. **Balance of spirit!**

I always considered it a privilege to participate in the development of my client's road to well-being! It gave me tremendous pride and honor to be able to interact in the process of someone's self-efficacy.

III

UNDERSTANDING EXERCISE

Exercise, activity requiring physical effort, carried out to sustain or improve health, fitness and well-being.

Fitness, the condition of being physically fit and healthy.

Health, the state of being free from illness or injury, a person's mental or physical condition.

Humans have survived for over 200,000 years based on our physical and mental capabilities. We were able to evolve based on both our mental and physical condition. Up until most recently and I mean two hundred years ago, humans required skills that were for the most part physical. Examples of this would be hunting skills and building skills. Physical effort was required for maintaining everything, there were no machines doing everything for us. Most jobs were labor based, building things by the power of the human body and mind. The survival of our tribal existence is a result of how strong and disciplined their warriors were. How skilled they became. Before the invention of the gun a warrior would have to be highly skilled at weapons, they most likely made themselves. There armies were as strong as their skill, strength and discipline. Today, Basic Training in the U.S. ARMY is 22 weeks, that's three months of grueling exercise and mental discipline. Potential soldiers are pushed to their physical and mental limits, it takes three months to discipline a person to become a soldier.

Greece, is the first known empire with evidence of exercise used for the purpose of Strength, Endurance and Speed. They, of course are the originators of the **Olympic games** which dates back to **776 BC.** It is only most recently in history, that people have exercised for the sole purpose of health and well-being. People used to sustain a high level of activity, which kept them fit and healthy and they only consumed the amount of food

26

needed to sustain their activity. They didn't over eat because the food wasn't readily available to them like it is today.

In the late 1890's, strength training was considered bad for you.

In 1936, Jack Lalane opens first modern era Gym in Oakland, California, and also designed many of modern day exercise machines, such as Leg extension.

Between 1927-1947, the Harvard fatigue lab was the first organization to advise both, Strength and endurance training for well-being.

In 1949, Jerry Morris makes the first Connection between Cardiovascular health and exercise.

In Early 1950s, the treadmill is invented for medical testing. Soon after is used to provide prisoners with a means of exercise!

Between 1950-1960, exercise was promoted as medicine. The health is Wealth belief. Very few people strength train.1953 Edmund Hillary summits Mt Everest. Not until the early 60s was the Treadmill marketed for in-home use. In 1960s, FAD diets became a craze.

In the 1970's, running became popular. Jim fix book Running appears on the New York times best sellers list and fuels the rise in Marathon participation. Organizations are founded and devoted to the science of exercise.

In 1972, Nike produces its first running shoe, the waffle sole shoe designed by Bill Bowerman co-founder of Nike.

In 1977, Body Building or you may call it weight training, became popular fueled by Arnold Schwarzenegger and his Documentary Pumping Iron. Joe Weider develops gyms, equipment and magazine oriented to exercise.

In 1980's, group fitness classes became popular. Jane Fonda introduced her series of best-selling Aerobic videos. Micheál Jordan became the most popular athlete in the world and promotes strength training.

In 1990's, more people began strength training. Yoga and Pilates type exercises became popular.

In 2000's, Exercise became a proven scientific benefit to health. Athletes depend on fitness trainers. Personal trainers become popular.

Ironically with all the advancements in technology and the presence of gyms, exercise fads, healthier foods, in home exercise equipment, humans have significantly more issues with obesity, health and wellbeing than they had a few hundred years ago.

Humans today are far less active and eat more than they need. We have become much less physically capable. Work habits have change to where more people are in chairs most of the work day. The human body has not evolved or change very much for that matter in the last thousands of years. In order to be healthy, we still require our bodies and mind to be active. On the other hand, our minds are evolving rapidly, and therein lies the problem. Our society is evolving toward humans being much less active. That's why a regular routine of some sort of activity is **vital** to your well-being. It's in our **DNA.** Everyone has a responsibility to themselves; to stay healthy and have vigor.

I realize for most people, figuring out how to exercise consistently is a difficult process. Its perceived as being burdensome. I think it's best to make exercise as simple as possible. Understanding the **principles** and **fundamentals** of exercise will give you a clearer picture as to what's involved in starting your pursuit. There are so many different ways that a person can exercise. it's a matter of choosing what's best for you and your life style.

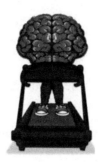

The Principles of Exercise:

1. **Individuality** complies with age, genetic ability, body type, muscle fibre type and mental state. It is best to find exercises that suits your individuality.
2. **Specificity** improves your ability in a specific activity. For instance, training for a marathon.
3. **Progression,** in order to reach your full capability, you have to progress slowly. it's like climbing a staircase that has 30 stairs, you have to be able to climb each level of stairs while maintaining your body positioning and breathing pattern. Strength and conditioning is not the same experience for everyone. Evolve at your own speed. The only thing that matters is that you in fact evolve. Adhere to your training and you will evolve.
4. **Overload**, in order to increase strength and endurance the resistance and intensity requires overload. If you can do 5 pushups, push yourself to do 10 and it will have a cascade of effect on your mind and body.
5. **Adaptation** over time helps adapt to a stimulus at a certain level. The first time you do an exercise that is an overload, your body will feel the result, also known as 'onset muscle sourness.' However, once you adapt to the stimulus change in intensity and time are needed for improvement.
6. **Recovery** is one of the most important aspects of exercise is recovery. Over use creates injury.

7. **Reversibility,** if you discontinue any activity or exercise over a period of time, your body will reverse and lose the gains it has achieved. Hence, muscle atrophy will occur.

These principles are the blueprints for exercise, the foundation in which any type of fitness activity is based on.

The Defining Fundamentals of Fitness Include,

1. **Muscular endurance,** doing as many push-ups as you possibly can.
2. **Muscular strength,** weight training, muscles begin to exert force.
3. **Cardiovascular endurance,** Aerobic exercise, long runs.
4. **Flexibility,** the ability to move any muscle through its full range of motion.
5. **Make a fitness program,** it shows entail how long, how often, and what type of activity you'd perform. The performance should be based on your goals and purpose.
6. **Co-ordination,** the ability to perform a movement smoothly and with control.
7. **Speed,** the maximum rate of contraction of a muscle.

All exercise should include a minimum of 10-20 minute warm up and cool down.

Deep breathing: Always exhale on exertion of energy, inhale when returning to original position. Proper breathing is one of the body's self-healing mechanisms. Before you start any exercise program, you should always consult a doctor.

Cardiovascular exercise, is any activity that raises your heart rate, and increases the health of the lungs and cardiovascular system, for instance running, biking, or rowing. Your maximum heart rate is 220 - your age. For instance, if you are 40 years old, your maximum heart rate would be 220-40 which equals 180. Tour target heart rate is 65-75% of that, which equals at a 70% calculation to be 126. In this example, this 40-year-old persons' fat burning zone would be 125-130 maximum. I used to do the talk test with my clients. Exercising at this level you should be able speak completely normal in this range of BPM. Monitoring your heart rate is important. Place two fingers on your wrist. Locate your pulse and time for 15 seconds and multiply by four to get your beats per minute (BPM).

Benefits of Cardiovascular Exercise:

1. Lowers blood pressure
2. Makes your heart stronger
3. Reduces depression and stress
4. Promotes a healthy vascular system
5. Increases blood flow
6. Increases bone density
7. reduces body fat

Anaerobic Exercise

Anaerobic Power: Rate at which work is done with an effective combination of force and speed.

Anaerobic Capacity: The total energy output during a specific period of time. Combines muscular strength, muscular endurance.

Agility: Speed or reaction resulting from a combination of co-ordination, balance and anaerobic power. The muscular system is vital to our well-being for so many reasons.

Muscle, a band or bundle of fibrous tissue in a human or animal body that has the ability to contract, producing in or maintaining the position of parts of the body. In essence every move your body produces are based on muscle. The following is a list of benefits of **muscle.**

Benefits of Muscle

1. Lowers blood sugar levels
2. Muscle makes bones stronger
3. Creates healthy joints and range of motion
4. Builds strength and endurance
5. Enhances state of mind and body

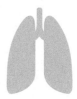

31

6. Helps reduce stress and depression.

and so much more. Muscle is the furnace of our bodies. It is responsible for how we metabolize what we consume. It gives you self-confidence. Muscle weighs twice the amount of Fat so if you gain muscle and lose fat at the same time, your bathroom scale will not give you a true picture of your body composition.

Different muscle fibres are responsible for particular movements. Some of muscle fibres are enlisted below.

1. **Slow Twitch Muscle Fibre,** used predominately for endurance training.
2. **Fast Twich Muscle Fibre,** used predominately for short bursts of strength, jumping activity.

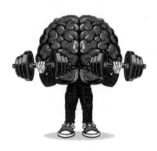

Muscle is the Foundation of the Human Body

Which now brings me to body types and how different body types should approach Exercise and Fitness. There are three distinct body composition types. Everyone fits into one of the following or you may have characteristics of more than one.

Endomorph

1. Larger bone structure with a large midsection and hips.
2. More fat throughout the Body.
3. Loses fat slow but gains fat fast.
4. Slow metabolism, more sedentary life style

Endomorphs, should be predominantly attentive to fat loss and strengthening of the cardiovascular system. Resistance training should be applied for the strengthening of muscles and joints as well as a consistent cardiovascular routine to increase metabolization. Endomorphs should be encouraged to increase their daily activities. Walk more and sit less. Endomorph is the hardest body type in terms of the level of difficulty in maintaining and managing weight gain.

Ectomorph

1. Tall and skinny.
2. Narrow shoulders and hips.
3. Smaller muscle in compared to bone size
4. Fast metabolism.
5. Difficult to gain and keep muscle

Ectomorphs, possess a very highly active metabolism and therefor it is more difficult to keep and gain muscle mass. A routine that focuses on Muscle Hypertrophy and gradual maximal strength gains should be the priority. The routine should focus less on cardio exercise for fat loss but more for maintenance and sustained health. One of my clients, many years ago was a true Ectomorph, a frustrated one at that. The client was a male around 30 years old and as skinny as you could imagine. He came to me because I was Training the owner of a restaurant and this guy was the Manager. That meant Free lunches for me and they were delicious. He on the other hand was very aggravated by his lack of not being able to gain muscle mass. He was never successful at gaining muscle mass with his past Trainers and he was in a state of frustration. I promised to help him. I Trained that poor guy harder than I have ever trained anyone. If he didn't almost vomit after every session I wasn't satisfied. On top of that, he was approximately 6'2 and 140 lbs., stark naked. I instructed him to eat as much healthy lean protein and tons of carbohydrates as much as he could and he did, he ate like a horse. It took about 6 months of that type of intensity for him to gain muscle. He was very committed to obtain his goals and I very much enjoyed working with him.

33

Mesomorph

1. Shoulders wider than hips.
2. Medium bone structure.
3. The body type of an Athlete.
4. Fast metabolizers.
5. Gaines Muscle fast and losses slowly with relatively less effort.
6. Efficient Fat burners

Mesomorphs, this is the body type that if maintained over your lifetime you will remain a Mesomorph. My body is a true Mesomorph and because of my commitment to maintaining my body to the highest level I have maintained the same waste size, 30 inches, my entire life. Exercise for this composition should be geared toward maximal gains in Muscular strength and endurance, cardiovascular endurance and agility training. Mesomorphs are compact and muscular. Your body type is basically a byproduct of your state of mind and your patterns of habit also Environment and Genetics have a great influence on your body composition.

I have witnesses entire transformation from one body type to another. I've seen over weight clients become thin, thin clients become muscular. I have seen it all! I can tell you without hesitation that it is possible to transform your body type. **Never** give up **hope**. You are not a prisoner to your **body type.**

It's Important to Understand the Different Types of Movement in the Body

1. **Isometric Movement,** a form of exercise involving the static contraction of a muscle without any movement to the angle of the joint". An Abdominal Plank Exercise would be an example.
2. **Isotonic Movement,** exercise in which opposing muscles contract and there is controlled movement, tension is constant while the lengths of the muscle changes. Push Ups, Squats and Biceps Curls are examples. Most common movements are **Isotonic.**
3. **Isokinetic Movement,** muscular action with a constant rate of movement. An example would be a stationary bike where there is

constant leg movement and the bike is providing the varied amount of resistance.

4. **Plyometric Movemen**t, exercise that focuses on **speed, agility, balance** and **power.** These include old school type movements such as Jumping Jacks, Speed Drills, Movement that involves your **own body weight.**

Exercise and **fitness** are not unlike any other form of **discipline.** Like dancing it takes time to cultivate and there are different **tempos, form** and **technique**, and all are essential. Both, Exercise and Dance require a regimented **stretching routine** to reach maximum goals and avoid injury, **stretching** is very important to the progress of overall health. I always spent at least 10-15 minutes at the end of every session to stretch my clients. It was most of my client's favorite part of the session. There are many publications available specifically on stretching. Rule of thumb is to stretch every muscle involved in the days exercise and its opposing muscle, if you exercise your chest then stretch your chest as well as your back and your Biceps and Triceps which are also the primary muscles involved in a chest press exercise. **Form** is **extremely** important when it pertains to stretching a specific muscle. Always move a muscle through its full range of motion.

Walking for exercise, another **underrated** activity. It is our mode of locomotion. I happen to think that walking is the best form of exercise. I'm talking about a purposeful walk not a browse at shop windows kind of walk. A walk with a swift pace and for the purpose of well-being. If you have never had a walking routine then slowly progress to a minimum of 30 minutes five times per week. The first week try walking as far as you can up to 30 minutes. If you feel like walking 15 mins is your maximum then start there and add 5 minutes every walk until you reach 30 minutes. My Father is 84 Years old and has been walking one hour every day for the last 25 years and plays several hours of tennis a week. He's able to do this because he has maintained his walking routine and he also has learned to enjoy stretching. I highly recommend building up to walking one hour per day.

Walking is proven to have improved mental health and decrease the chances of Alzheimer.

The benefits of walking are the following:

1. Walking for 30 minutes a day is a great way to maintain weight loss. Walking is one of the most effective ways to burn body fat.
2. Change of environment. Strengthens bones, reduces stress.
3. Boosts muscular endurance and strength.
4. Requires minimal equipment.
5. You can walk anywhere. it's an activity you can rely on.
6. Easy to initiate.
7. Choose climbing stairs whenever possible.

If you have a smart phone or any other step tracking device, I highly recommend counting steps. Between 5 and 7 thousand steps a day is a good target. Counting steps can be very rewarding. It is a confirmation of activity, a measured goal.

Measured goal, is very effective to have a measurable, Visual confirmation of your achievements. Step counters are very effective. My first-year training at Ballys. Total Fitness I was training a very high-profile client and his then girlfriend. His girlfriend was younger and was very fit. He was not so fit in fact he was 20 pounds overweight. She was a great motivator for him and over time he achieved great results. When I stopped working at Ballys. I lost contact with both of them. Ten years later I was sitting having a coffee at my local coffee shop and guess who's there. It was outside on the patio and he was sitting in the corner on his computer snacking on two muffins and a scone. He hadn't seen me yet so I spent a little time watching him before I went over and said hello. He didn't take hie eyes off his computer and he had eaten these two large muffins. He also was not the fit person I had left at Ballys. I thought for a moment before I moseyed over to his table, I was thinking how I should approach him, what should I say. I'm a pretty blunt and straight to the point person. I went over to his table and got his eyes off his computer. He looked at me and I sat down. Hey, how you doing blah blah blah and I say 'WHAT THE F—K is going on with you.' I could see that he was embarrassed sitting there eating all that junk food. I said when I left you were very fit. His reply was that he had grown his business to become the largest of its kind in the world and I have no time to work out lately. I spoke the truth to him and told him that he looked terrible. He looked sick. I was very fond of him. I asked him what was he going to do about his state. He wasn't interested in weight training anymore and I wasn't after a client, I was too busy any way. He turned the table on me and asked me what I suggest. I asked him where he lived and worked. He lived in my neighbourhood just outside the City and worked right Downtown, probably a 10 mile walk there and back. It was the beginning of summer so I suggested that he walk to and from work every day until it gets cold again. I thought it a long shot but you never know. He thought for a moment and said WOW that's a great idea. We shook hands and I asked him to promise me that he would do it. He was the type of person that could keep a promise. I ran into him several months later and sure enough he was still walking to and from work and he was trim again all from just walking. He thanked me and said that it was the best exercise he had ever done and while walking he was able to think clearer.

Ground Reaction Force, is the force exerted by the ground on a body in contact with it. This refers to gravity exerting force on your body. This is relevant in regard to posture. Pay very close attention to your posturing and gait while walking as incorrect posture can lead to joint issues. I used to tell my clients to imagine that a string at the top their head was pulling them up. Every time your foot leaves the ground while walking has a ground reaction force. The more your body leaves the ground the greater the compression on your body. Walking has a very low ground reaction force on your body, where as a sport like Tennis or Basketball have much larger force on your body. The force on your body while walking actually promotes stronger bones. It is highly important to make sure that your shoes are a good fit and support your gait properly. The best thing to do is to go to a reliable running shoe store that can analyze your gait and suggest a proper shoe. Every shoe brand has a different fit and feel.

It became my mantra, that every person I trained should start a walking routine. I ended up walking 6-7 hours a day. I was not walking my clients I was helping them form the habit which in this case was walking. I would consider walking to be the best approach to the start of a fitness program. Find a walking partner if possible. When I walk, I think. Walking for me has become a pleasure and something I do daily with my three dogs.

Sought After Benefits from Exercise

1. Management and treatment of injuries and health issues.
2. Improves co-ordination
3. Improved health in general.
4. Reduced risk of skeletal injury; breaking bones.
5. Increased ease of movement and performance of daily tasks.
6. Greater mind and body awareness.
7. Increased enjoyment of being physical.
8. Increase in energy level.
9. Increase in muscle mass.
10. Fat loss
11. Enhanced appearance; Muscle tone.
12. Improve confidence and self-image.

COMPONENTS OF A WORK OUT

1. Mental preparation, visualization
2. Cardiovascular warm up (minimum 20 minutes)
3. Strength training
4. Cardiovascular cool down (5-10 minutes stretch)
5. Stretching
6. Maintain a strong energy after your workout allow yourself to be more relaxed

Benefits of Stretching

1. Reduced stress on joints and muscle tissue
2. Lowers risk of back pain
3. Improved balance and muscular awareness
4. Increased mind and body awareness
5. Increased blood supply to joints and muscle
6. Decreased risk of injury

I can't stress enough the importance of **warm up** and **cool down. The underlying rational** for warm up and cool down is based upon the fact that various body systems require a certain amount of time to adapt to a change in physical stress on the body from an increase of physical activity.

Visualization, can be very effective in inspiring a workout. I always premeditated a workout that I was going to have, it gave me a sense of excitement a goal ready to be acted on.

The most critical period for anyone starting an exercise program is the first **3-6 months.** There is a much greater chance of long-term commitment to fitness after the 6 months period. It is completely normal to have lapses from time to time it's inevitable. Try to acquire a support system, friends family members that essentially become your cheerleaders.

Factors Influencing Adherence

Decreased program adherence is related to the following,

1. Presence of health issues.
2. Poor nutritional/Health habits.
3. Lack of education toward health.
4. high body fat.
5. Low self-motivation.
6. Inactive lifestyle
7. Perceived lack of time
8. Social relationship issues
9. Spouse or Partner non supportive

Increased program adherence is related to the following:

More than anything, adherence is driven by results, Positive feedback from others has a tremendous positive effect on adherence.

1. Healthy lifestyle habits
2. Support from spouse or partner
3. Highly self-motivated
4. Educated on health

39

5.   Realization and belief in health benefits

Strength Training Guidelines

Exercise selection

Choose exercises that you find enjoyable, be sure to include all the major muscle groups in your choice, including

1.   Back, Resistance band row.
2.   Chest, Exercise ball chest dumbbell press.
3.   Shoulders, Lateral raise with resistance band.
4.   Biceps, Bicep curl with resistance band.
5.   Triceps, Triceps dips.
6.   Calves, Ball Calf raises.
7.   Legs Ball Squats.

Always do a warm up set with low weight and high repetition to prepare the muscle for potentially more heavier sets.

Movement Speed

Slow controlled movement produces maximum results. When you are strength training and overload is involved try to feel every muscle used during a specific exercise. Slowing down the speed or increasing the speed have different effects. I usually split up workouts to where some are fast and others slower. Average most effective speed is 2-3 seconds to raise a weight and 3-4 seconds to lower the weight.

Circuit Training

Going from one exercise to another without rest in between. Involves endurance, resistance and aerobic exercise.

Form Proper form in regard to strength training involves isolated movement, proper spine alignment, proper breathing pattern and full range of motion.

12 WEEK EXERCISE PROGRAM

PHASE 1 (1 - 3 WEEKS)

Goals, to learn proper **Form** and introduce basic fundamental exercises. Start a walking program.

Training Do 1 set low intensity high repetition body weighted exercises, Focus on technique and form. Do as many forms of Correct push-ups as possible and add one per day on strength training days. Also include lunges, do as many as possible for both legs then add one per leg on strength training days.

Cardio Walk with intensity for 15-20 minutes. You should be able to talk normally during your walk don't push yourself (YET) to where it is difficult to breathe.

Weekly schedule, X represents including that activity in your day's

routine.

	Sunday	Monday	Tuesday	Wednesday	Thursday	Friday	Saturday
Walking	Rest Day	X	X	X	X		X
Training	Rest Day	X		X		X	
Stretching	Rest Day	X	X	X	X	X	X

PHASE 2 (3-6 WEEKS)

Goals, to gradually increase intensity and duration of exercise.

Training, do 2 sets of both, your maximum number of push-ups and lunges, Add squats and bird dog exercise. Rest of 1-1/2 minutes after each set.

Cardio, walk with more intensity and greater distance. Increase to minimum 0f 30-40 minutes. Change your route and include some hills and or stairs.

PHASE 3 (6-9 WEEKS)

Goals, to maintain Intensity.

Training, to maintain 2 sets of your maximum amount per exercise. Add an abdominal plank exercise for 15 seconds and add 5 seconds. Each training day. Rest of 1-1/2 minutes per set

Cardio, to maintain walking routine with same intensity

PHASE 4 (9-12 WEEKS)

Goals Increase Intensity

Training Add a third set. Do 3 sets of all exercises to your maximum amount each. 30 second rest between sets.

Cardio, increase walking time to 45-60 mins. Every 10 mins of walking, walk as fast as you can for 30-60 seconds. Start carrying either a back pack filled with 5-10 pounds or hand weights that are 2-5 pounds. Make sure that you rest between sets. There should be a rest week between phase 2 and 3.

Exercise Selection

Body Weighted Exercises

Squat: Stand straight with feet shoulder width apart, flex your stomach muscles and lower yourself like you were sitting in a chair. Bend your knees keeping your upper body straight until your upper legs are parallel to the floor. Don't allow your foot to come too far over your big toe. Great lower body movement for strength, endurance, co-ordination and flexibility. Variation is a squat jump.

Lunges: Stand straight and tall with your feet hip width apart. Take a giant step forward and plant your heel on the ground your upper leg should be parallel to the floor and your right shin is vertical. Press into your right heel to return to natural position. Repeat with opposite leg. Again, your knee should only slightly be over your big toe. Great for co-ordination, strength, endurance and flexibility. Variations are lunge jumps.

Push-ups: Get into a push-up position with your hands under your shoulders with your feet at hip width apart and parallel to each other. Align hips with shoulders and have your back in a natural position, not completely flat. Flex your stomach and think about bringing your belly button in toward your spine. Head position should be your ears in line with your shoulder. Lower your body toward the floor until your upper arm is parallel to the ground. Push through your hands to return to beginning position. Count 2-3 seconds to go down and 3-4 seconds to come up. A variation is on your knees. Great exercise for muscular strength, endurance and stabilization. Recruits several muscle groups. **Push -up challenge: Do 5-10 push-ups every two hours, every day for three weeks!**

Abdominal Plank: Lying face down on the floor put yourself in a plank position. Forearms and toes are on the floor. Elbows are directly under the shoulder and arms are facing forward. Flex your core muscles and hold. Make sure you breathe through the exercise. Your back should be in a neutral position and be sure to keep your hips up. Great for strengthening core muscles.

Bird Dog: Kneel on a soft surface with your knees hip width apart and your Hands under your shoulders. Be sure to flex your core muscles. Extend your arm straight out in front of you and at the same time extend the opposite leg until it is straight. Repeat for opposite leg. Great balance and stabilizer exercise. Works back stabilizers as well.

On completion of this 12-week program, your body is known ready for more. If you choose to repeat this 12-week program and find it challenging that's perfectly o.k. however if you wish to pursue a resistant training program, I recommend an **Exercise Ball** and a **Resistance Band.** Refer to the resistant training section for exercises for each muscle group.

43

FEEL GOOD LOOK GOOD LIVE GOOD

RE-CONNECT

IV

EMILLIO

Several years ago, I was working out at a local Gym that is part of a large chain. It was the first time in quit awhile that I had a membership at a gym, I was boxing a lot and I was exercising mostly at home so I really didn't need a gym. I was also not Personal Training at that time. For me going to a gym is like a fine tailor going to a boutique clothing store, you're in your element. Constantly observing how people incorrectly exercise and all the nuances in a Gym environment. I'm always on the lookout for potential clients even though I wasn't looking, it's in my nature. I would always in a very soft approach help people if I could or suggest different things to them. Most people were receptive and appreciated the advice.

The Gym had a very active Personnel Training Dept with some very good and some not so good Trainers. The good trainers were always busy. One Trainer in particular was in my radar. I would describe him as about 27 years old 5'11 inches tall and about 250 pounds of bulky muscle and no flexibility, He didn't look very fit... I had been watching him for months. Paying close attention to his workout patterns and how often he was training. On several occasions I watched him train his clients. He was always given the clients that got a free session with their membership and had no intention or capacity to become a client. His skills were not very honed. He had no idea how to communicate with individuals he was training. He was very mechanical. After several months of my detective work, I approached him.

I had decided that I wanted to help this person and I knew I could. There was something about him. All the experience and knowledge I had acquired over so many years was yearning to be put into practice. I was like a mad scientist. I wanted to use this poor guy in an experiment that I had thought up. I wanted to pick someone in the gym and transform them. I walked up to him and told him that I would like to have a conversation with him. He

45

said yes and we went into one of the offices. I told him that I had been watching him for a while and that I wanted to help him. To my surprise he wasn't all that shocked. I explained my background in regard to being a well-established Trainer. Then I proceeded to explain to him how I instinctively knew how I could help him. Emilio was extremely sensitive, respectful, and receptive to help. He didn't look the part and he didn't speak the jargon. He was bulking up and lifting very heavy weight because he was insecure. His mind and body were not jelling and I knew it. As I said I hadn't been training and I wanted to apply all my past experience and knowledge and change this young man. I was actually very excited. I was going to the gym more to see him than to train myself. He was such a sweet guy. He just needed some fine tuning. He needed to change his whole approach to fitness and himself.

After our hour conversation, I told him that the next time I'm in the gym would be in two days and that we should start a program he agreed and we arranged a time. I was grateful that this opportunity had presented itself. After devoting a great deal of thought I decided that I was going to test out a theory that had thought up. I had come across many people on my own journey that were into the physical aspect of fitness but didn't really understand what the mental aspect of it was or they just were not aware of it. I wanted to teach Emilio both right from the start. My intention was to strip Emilio down to the bare bones, start from scratch. A blank canvas.

When I arrived at the gym as per our arranged plan he was waiting and eager to get started. No chatting just right to work. I had him go on the treadmill, I wanted to see how his cardio was. It wasn't very good, all that bulky muscle weight him down and thus he had no endurance. Was no surprise to me. He did 10 mins at a low level and was tired. I suggested 30 mins of cardio a day and absolutely no weight training. The next exercise I had him do was to see how many **forms of correct** push-ups he could do. He did 12. For the next three weeks his program was 30 mins of cardio a day and to add a push up every day. He kinda looked at me weird but I assured him this is what he needed. At the same time, I asked him about his life style his habits. He was a big meat eater. I asked him if he would be willing to try other forms of protein that didn't have as much saturated fat, so he started eating more fish, salmon in particular. He was 100%

committed. The reason for that was, he wanted to be challenged. I knew it, and so did he. I told him that in 3 weeks, we would make further changes, but sticking with the plan was a must. What he didn't know, is that I was starting to get into his head. I'm actually very good at it, it's my specialty. I wanted to find out what his life was like so I could work toward him a having a good feeling about himself. I purposely completely altered his routine and made him do exercises that he had never done before. I knew that he needed to be less bulky. At the same time, I wanted to increase his speed and work on his agility. I instinctively knew that Emilio had a different visual of himself in his mind than what the physicality presented.

Three weeks later Emilio had done his cardio every day and could now do 40 push-ups. Every time I saw him there after I would spend 15-20 minutes talking to him. He was such a sweet sole that it made me feel good to validate him, encourage him. I now instructed him to do as many squat jumps as he could. A squat jump is a plyometric agility exercise where you bend your knees until your upper leg is parallel to the ground and then propel yourself vertically as high as you can, making sure your knee does not go past your big toe when you land. Emilio did 7.

I told him to know add 10 mins to his cardio do the 40 push-ups and to add the squat jumps and add one per day. So now he's doing 40 mins of cardio 40 pushups and the squat jumps. The best part is that Emilio is evolving, he now is talking about becoming vegan and articulating how different he already feels. Whenever we spoke I always gave him a hint a day on the secretes to working more as a Trainer. What important questions to ask potential clients. What red flags to look for.

Another three weeks went by, and I had now seen Emilio three to four times a week and we always engaged each other. Now he was doing 40 push-ups, 30 squat jumps and 40 mins of cardio daily. Time to add another 10 mins to his cardio and now I instructed him to do Sprints. I set up two cones about 25 feet apart from each other and he had to run between them for 30 seconds with a 30 secs rest. He did his first one and as I suspected he was way outta breath. I added the 30 second sprint and he had to add 5 seconds per day for the next three weeks. After six weeks Emilio is starting to show very encouraging progress. Every three weeks I added 10 mins to his cardio and another body weighted exercise.

Week 9: Jumping Jacks were added and Emilio did 20 and he had to once again add one jumping jack per day. Now he was doing 40 pushups, 30 squat jumps, a minute and a half of sprints and one hour of cardio. This young man's energy was in a state of metamorphosis in nine weeks he had shed a significant amount of body fat but more importantly he was starting to feel really good about himself which was also starting to have a spillover effect in regard to his skills at acquiring clients. His energy level had increased and his personality started shining through. He was now able to teach what he was living. He was now doing 2 sets for each exercise.

Week 12: Walking lunges are added. Emilio did 25 and had to add one per workout. Know he's doing, 40 lunges, 40 pushups, 30 squat jumps, a minute and a half of sprints and now I instructed him to one do 20 mins of intense cardio, meaning he increased the speed on the treadmill to where he was running fast for 20 minutes. He was now doing three sets for each exercise.

After 12 weeks, Emilio has a constant smile on his face. He completely had transformed his body and mind. It was actually amazing to witness such a dramatic change in a person. Emilllio over the next 6 months had become one of the Top Trainers and had altered his life in every respect. His confidence was beaming like a bright light. He was now a well-rounded fit person able to do anything physically he desired. Other members of the gym that new Emilio were approaching me and communicating how wonderful it was to see Emilio so bright. It obviously made me very fulfilled to have had the opportunity to help Emilio. It made me a bigger person.

V

METABOLISM

Metabolism, is "The Chemical process that occurs within a living organism in order to maintain life." An efficient metabolism is essential to Well-Being. It's where we get our energy and power from. Metabolization creates energy.

Energy production on a cellular level

What does the human body use as energy at the cellular level?

1. The ATP system of energy

A molecule called ATP (Adenosine Triphosphate), is chemically broken down to release energy. ATP is stored within all the cells of the body, particularly in Muscle Cells. ATP is formed with the energy release from food, and is the most immediately used source of energy for all cellular functions and muscle contractions. The food that you eat is actually what produces ATP and what gives you energy. The three main components are,

1. Fat (Fatty Acids), used for energy stored as body fat.
2. Carbohydrates (Glucose), used as energy and stored as glycogen in the muscles.
3. Protein (Amino Acids), essential for the growth and repair of tissues.

ATP supplies energy to your body for up to 10 seconds

2. Anaerobic Glycolysis

This system of energy relies on ATP but also utilizes glucose, and glycogen which is stored in muscles.

Anaerobic Glycolysis supplies energy for an average of up two minutes

3. Aerobic Glycolysis

This system relies on a small amount of ATP, but prominently breaks down Blood Sugar using oxygen. After approximately 20 minutes, the body begins to use predominant fat stored as energy. This system of energy introduces oxygen for sustained amounts of exercise. A long run would be an Aerobic exercise.

After 20 minutes of high intensity exercise, your body switches to an aerobic system.

It's very similar to a car that has an automatic gear shift. Every time you change the gears, the car accelerates faster and becomes more efficient with having to put less stress on the engine. Similarly, a car requires gas in order for it to move. Humans require food for the same reason. Plants receive energy from sunlight. Every living thing needs a source of energy to survive.

Rapid powerful   1/4 mile sprint   Jogging for 20 mins

Bursts of energy

(0-10) sec

————————————I———————————————I———————————————

ATP   Anaerobic ATP, Blood Sugar.   Aerobic Fat Burn

What effects your metabolism negatively?

1. Age.
2. Genetics.
3. Lack of Sleep.
4. Lack of activity.
5. Being overweight.
6. Unhealthy Food.

What effects your metabolism positively?

1. Exercise.
2. Lean muscle mass.
3. Proper sleep.
4. Healthy Food.
5. Staying hydrated.
6. Managing stress.
7. Lean muscle mass. It helps strengthen the immune system.

Food Consumption Process

Digestion is the breakdown of large insoluble food molecules, into small, water-soluble molecule, so that they can be absorbed into the blood plasma. The digestive system is very sensitive and energy consuming. In fact, 5-10% of your body's energy is used in digestion.

Digestion Process

Molecules absorbed into blood - Transportation

To Active Cells (site of energy production) - For immediate use or storage!

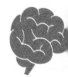

How should you improve digestion?

1. If you have digestive issues refer to **FODMAP** for wiser choices of food.

2. High Fibre Foods. For instance, **Metamucil** is a terrific source of fibre.

3. Scheduled eating.

4. Drink Water. Water is vital for digestion.

5. Exercise.

6. Manage stress. Stress has a large effect on your digestion.

7. High fatty foods take a longer time to digest using more water and energy.

There is a lot of chatter out there in regard to calories, and it has become yet another buzz word that is used to manipulate people into buying beliefs in 'Calorie free this and Calorie free that.' It's all very confusing. Let's get to the bottom of what calorie really is.

Calorie is "The energy needed to raise the temperature of 1 gram of water through a temperature of 1 degree Celsius." Eating creates energy. It works the same way as the locomotive trains would use wood burning steam engines. The team of workers in the engine room had to constantly throw on wood logs to keep the fire hot enough to create steam. Instead of throwing small pieces of wood, they used to throw in large and thick pieces of wood that took longer to burn. The log in this example represents a well-balanced healthy meal.

Where do calories come from?

1. Fat: Contains 9 calories per gram.

2. Carbohydrates: Contains 4 calories per gram.

3. Protein: Contains 4 calorie per gram.

4. Alcohol: Contains 7-9 calorie per gram.

YOU ARE WHAT YOU EAT

I have always advised my clients to think about what I call the 'Three w's of eating.'

1. When are you eating is closely related to what time of day are you're eating.

2. Why are you eating relates to consuming proper food requirements for your energy needs.

3.   What are you eating. It is essential to eat appropriate foods to sustain
     energy needs.

The average daily calorie requirements

Male: 1400-1800 calories.

Female: 1200-1400 calories.

How should one increase caloric expenditure?

1. Increase muscle mass.

2. Increase activity level. If you sit a lot all day get up and walk around every 30 minutes.

3. Healthy food. Eat meals that combine all the food groups.

4. Cut back on high sugar and saturated fatty foods.

5. Cardiovascular Exercise.

"Your calories expenditure in, should equal the calorie expenditure out."

Try to eat foods that have less ingredients. If the food has more than 5-10 ingredients, then it's better to stay miles away from consuming that food. Try making fresh food choices whenever possible. Refer to the **Glycemic Index** for foods to analyze how quickly it helps convert sugar into energy. Limit your food intake that is high in saturated fat.

Saturated fat, a type of fat that is found in:

1. Butter.

2. Meat.

3. Vegetable Fat.

4. Egg Yolks.

How to decrease your caloric intake

1. Count your Caloric intake.

2. Use less condiments and sauces.

3. Don't drink high caloric drinks.

4. Limit sugar in tea and coffee.

5. Try to cook your own food as much as possible.

6. Limit junk food in your house.

7. Use smaller plates. Smaller plates will eventually help you having smaller portions of meal.

8. Eat more vegetables.

9. Eat slowly and in a relaxed state.

10. Limit the intake of high sugar carbohydrates.

11. Eat whole fruits.

12. Limit Alcohol intake.

13. Swap unhealthy foods for healthier choices.

14. Consuming excess calories means you're eating more than your body actually requires.

Your **basic metabolic rate** is the number of calories your body uses to sustain life and perform all essential functions of the body. The formula to figure out your rate is based on the most reliable source to date; The Miffen-St Jeor equation.

Male = 10 x weight (kg) + 6.25 x your height (cm) - 5 x age (years) + 5

Female = 10 x weight(kg) + 6.25 x your height(cm) - 5 x age (years) - 1

Water intake is integral for well-being. 11/2 - 2 litres a day is the recommended amount.

1. Blood is 85% water.

2. Brain is 75% water.

3. Lungs are 90% water.

4. Skin is 80% water.

5. Bones are 24% water.

6. Muscle is 75% water.

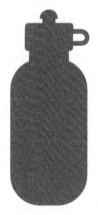

Benefits of drinking water

1. Prevents dehydration which can cause confused thinking.

2. Prevents the body from over exhaustion.

3. Prevents kidney stones.

4. Your cells rely on water for well-functioning.

5. Maximizes physical capabilities.

6. Lack of water affects energy and brain function.

7. Necessary for proper digestion.

8. Decreases inflammation.

9. Aids in weight loss.

Your body uses water in two ways. Intra cellular water is the water within the cell over which cell function relies on. Extra cellular water is the water in your blood that your body relies on, for organ functionality, muscle movement, and all other bodily function. Intracellular water makes up for 70% of all the water in your body. Decrease Your amount of sodium intake. Too much salt actually draws water out of your cells. Limit the intake of the following high sodium foods. You could do that by avoiding the following consumables.

1. Fast Food.
2. Salty Snacks.
3. Frozen and processed foods.
4. Processed meat.
5. Salty soups.
6. Most boxed Food.
7. The recommended daily amount of salt is 1500-2000 mg per day.

Limit amounts of the following foods

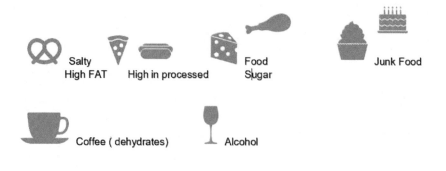

Salty
High FAT   High in processed   Food Sugar   Junk Food

Coffee (dehydrates)   Alcohol

7 Steps to Optimal Performance and maintaining Well-being

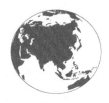

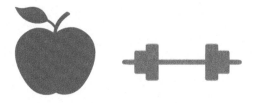

Take care of your environment   **Eat Healthy Food**   **Exercise**

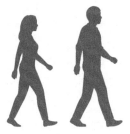

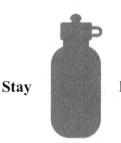

Walk   **Stay**   **Hydrated**

Manage your time   **Manage**   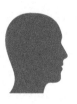   **stress**

Hormones are like tiny little messengers that are chemically activated and travel in the Bloodstream to either your organs, or tissue. They have a great effect on your overall health and well-being.

Hormones Effect the following functions:

1. Development.
2. Growth.
3. Metabolism.
4. Reproduction.
5. Sexual Function.
6. Mental state.
7. Energy Levels.

Hormones are extremely powerful and can change your life in either a positive or a negative way. It only takes a very small amount of hormones to have a huge effect on your entire body.

How do hormones effect your well-being?

Serotonin, also known as the mood hormone. You could do the following to enhance the levels of Serotonin in the body.

1. Spend time outdoors.

2. Minimal sun exposure.

3. Consuming healthy foods such as Oatmeal, Salmon, Brown Rice, Nuts, and whole grain breads.

4. Walking outdoors.

5. Hiking, and enjoying nature.

Endorphins, also known as the anti-stress and pain hormone can be elevated by doing the following.

1. Regular Exercise.

2. Vigorish activity.

3. Smiling and laughing.

4. Consuming Dark Chocolate.

5. Dancing.

6. Celebrating Life

7. Walking.

Dopamine, also known as the reward hormone can be elevated by the following:

1. Being Disciplined. For instance, finishing a task.

2. Getting adequate and quality sleep.

3. Being creative.

4. Self-Care such as a massage or a therapeutic activity.

5. A hobby.

6. Playing a sport.

Oxytocin, the-love-feel-good hormone can be increased in the body by incorporating the following activities in your life, some of which are listed below.

1. Having a dog or cat.

2. Music.

3. Watching a good film.

4. Human contact and touch.

5. Random acts of kindness.

6. Yoga.

7. Being complimentary.

8. Being appreciative and forgiving toward others.

VI

THE JOHN MUIR TRAIL

In 1979, I was living in New York City, studying acting at the Lee
rasberg Theatre School, which at the time was the best institute in the world
study acting. Actors such as Al Pacino and Robert De Niro, were heavily
fluenced by Lee Strasberg. New York City in the late 70's and early 80's,
is in the influence of a cultural revolution of every kind. It was an amazing
perience to live in the city and see the culture, forming right before your
es. I witnessed the birth of Graffiti, Break Dancing and Rap. It was all alive
the streets of the City and I was living the life as an actor. New York was
huge learning experience for me. I was 18 years old when I moved there
d it made me grow very quickly.

My first day in New York was quite an exciting one. I was on a lunch
eak from school, so I decided to walk down the street to Union Square Park,
hich at the time was referred to as needle park. It was infested with drugs
d victims of drugs. I sat on a Bench and started eating my lunch, a Sandwich
om the Deli. As I'm taking my first bite into my first sandwich in NYC, this
g guy comes, walking over to me and asks me if I want to buy some drugs.
eplied no and he then said that I was sitting on his bench and that I needed
get off. I really didn't know what to do, so I got up with my sandwich in
nd and as, I leave, this guy kicks me, right in the Crotch and tells me to
ver come back into the Park. It felt like I was going to die, it was probably
e closest a male could come, to having an understanding of the pain of child
th. He was my welcoming committee to New York. I knew right at that
oment that I needed to be very careful This was a ruthless place. After living
the City for several years, I decided at the urging of my teachers to get out
Los Angeles and study Film acting. I thought it to be a good idea and started
anning my departure by car.

Approximately two days before I was scheduled to leave, I was in Central
rk and by pure chance, met my future wife. I did not know it at the time but
turned out to be true. I met her in Central Park, she was crying on a bench,

so I went over to her. I had seen her a few times before and this was the perfe
opportunity. I approached her and we started talking. She was crying becau
her previous boyfriend had committed suicide. We instantly connected. T
most amazing thing actually happened was the Late Comic Genius, Rob
Williams, playing the Saxophone with a case in front of him for tips. He w
wearing a black jacket and a hat and did not want to be noticed. He w
playing for us on our first meeting. We respected that but however, we kne
who he was. Turns out that he was practicing the Saxophone for a role ir
movie called 'Moscow On The Hudson.' It was one of many amazi
experiences, living in the Big Apple. Anyway, I asked her out on a date th
night, and it was my last night in New York. I had already packed up n
things and loaded everything I owned, which was not much for my litt
Volkswagen Scirocco. She said yes, and we went to see a James Bond mov
called, Octopussy and had dinner at the famous hamburger joint called '
Clarkes.' I did not want to leave without her. After one date, and one night
asked her if she would be interested in moving to Los Angles. I was drivi
back to Toronto to spend a month with my Family and then, driving all t
way across the United States from Toronto to Los Angeles, approximate
2500 miles. She ended up flying to Toronto and with my little sister, we
got into the car and Drove to LA LA land.

By the time we arrived in L. A., and after a very long and eventful driv
it was time for me to start looking for a place to live. Hats off, when Donn
this girl I had fallen in love with, decided to stay and live in L.A. We leas
an apartment in the Westwood neighbourhood of L.A., where UCLA
located. I fell in love with Los Angeles and had the time of my life with n
girlfriend who is now my wife of 39 years.

After living in Los Angeles for a couple of years, we decided to mo
back to New York, closer to Donna and my families A couple of years lat
with our now, one-year-old baby, we left New York to live in Toronto.

I hadn't been to Los Angeles in several years and my friend Mark w
now living there. We had befriended one another working on a T.V. sho
together in 1980. His career as an actor was taking off. I missed L.A. and
in March 1987, I went to visit him. That's when the tradition of working o
and hiking in the different areas around L.A. began. Los Angeles has fantas

places to hike, some of them are very challenging. Every year in March, I would visit Mark and every year we would do something physically challenging. We started Mountain Biking on some extreme paths. The Back Bone Trail in the Santa Monica Mountains is an example. You're in the middle of L.A. but if you didn't know it, you would think you were in the Amazon Jungle. For many years, we did that trail and not without falls and injuries. On one occasion, myself, Mark, and another friend Eric were on the trial, and Eric got a flat tire about half way through the trail without a spare tube. We tried to Mcgyver it with chewing gum but it didn't work. He ended up having to walk his bike the rest of the trail while Mark and I rode down the rest of the way. At the end of the Trail is Will Rogers State Park, the old house where Will Rogers had lived. It's a Beautiful Place. It took Eric two hours to walk the trail, while we rested and tanned. At the same time, we started climbing any rock wall that looked climbable.

Eventually, and for many years, we started camping in Joshua Tree State Park. A place for serious hikes and climbs. It is a place that attracts serious climbers. It is in my opinion, the most peaceful place I have experienced in my entire life. There is an energy in the desert that provokes peace and the silence is blissful.

In 2007, we decided to really start challenging ourselves, we booked a trip to hike, 'The Jhon Muir Trail,' in Northern California, and finished with summiting of Mount Whitney, which at 14,505 feet, that makes it the tallest mountain in the continental United States. The hike itself was a 211-mile hike with some of the hardest Switch Backs around. A Switch Back in hiking terms is a trail that cuts sharply in one direction to the other while going up a very steep mountainside. It's used by hikers in order not to have to go straight up the Mountain, which would be much more difficult. We signed up and gave our deposits to the adventure company that was setting up the trip. It was cataloged as being one of the most difficult hikes that the travel company offered, and they arranged adventures all over the World National Geographic, calling it one of the top ten trails on the planet.

The Hike was to commence in September 2007, which meant that we had to start working out. Mark arrived in Toronto in June. We had two months to train, buy our equipment, and mentally prepare. We trained every day, except one rest day per week, for two months. We trained harder than I have ever trained. I think that was probably when I was the fittest, I have ever been. We were Boxing, doing sprints up the steep hills, skipping and resistance training to the point of exhaustion. It was both, our mission to be as capable as possible for our Hike.

The fun part was going to the Mountain climbing Store and picking out our equipment. Back Packs, Head Lamps, clothing and all the other essentials required for a three-Week hike. The most important item of all were the Hiking Boots. You literally have to try on ten pairs in order to get the right fit and I did. We decided that we would buy our boots and to work them in we would walk from my house to Lake Ontario. It's a 15 mile walk in new boots I had blisters everywhere and I remember being exhausted by the time we arrived back to my house. I think it took us 8 hours.

September was approaching very quickly and the realization of what was before me started to set in. Mark and I were guests on a very popular Radio Show. We were invited to talk about our trip and summiting Mount Whitney which was in two weeks from that date. Mark had returned to L.A., and a week later, I arrived. It was very hard for me to leave my family and Dogs As I did every time, I left home on a trip, I told my wife that I would see her soon, giving hugs and kisses. Los Angeles was experiencing a heat Wave and it was 110 degrees Fahrenheit. I arrived only a couple of days before our departure. Toronto was only 80 degrees that's a 30-degree difference in Temperature. It was barely tolerable in Los Angeles.

The day quickly arrived and our first destination was Fresno California where we were meeting up with the other people on the trip and the guides who were leading us on the trail. It was even Hotter in Fresno. It was so hot you could not go outside for more than ten minutes. We arrived at the Motel early that afternoon. That evening was the scheduled meeting to discuss all the protocols and rules for the trip and to get to know each other. There were ten other people and three guides. It took us a couple of hours to go over all the safety rules and chat about our route. Then, off we went to bed so we could wake up early the next morning to start our Big Adventure.

We woke up at six am sharp, had breakfast at seven o clock, and then loaded our gear into a large van that accommodated everyone and started our

ree-hour drive to Florence. We arrived at the lake where we met with the
rse packer and mule handlers to offload all the gear. We then boarded a
rry that transported us across the Lake. The first day's hike was a six-mile
ke along the beautiful banks of the San Joaquin River, so to connect us with
e Jhon Muir Trail. The trail Leeds through the Sierra Nevada Mountain
nge passing through Kings Canyon and Sequoia National Parks. Stunning
ountain peak views, waterfalls, and amazing flower-filled meadows that
oked like they were right out of the Wizard Of Oz. During the day we hiked
d at night we ate at Camp Fire dinners and had a good conversation and
en off to our tents for some needed sleep.

Waking in the morning in the wilderness is a very special Time. Instead
all the habits and responsibilities that you are attached to at home, in the
lderness, it's just you and Nature. No City Noise, Leaf Blowers and all the
her annoying elements of City Life. When you're in the middle of nowhere
e only sound you hear is the sound of silence and yourself, the buzz of the
orld. There is a very certain energy that exists in Nature that has been
moved from urban areas that are concrete jungles. There is peace,
nquility an appreciation for life and all living creatures. It's a feeling of
ing a part of something much larger. The bigger picture.

On the Fourth morning of the hike, I woke up early and decided to go,
d look for a good place for my morning ritual. Going to the bathroom
esn't exist, nature is the bathroom and it takes few, getting used to it. I
lked pretty far before I realized, I didn't know where I was, I had not paid
uch attention to where I was, there was so much beauty around me and I
ded up getting completely lost in the middle of nowhere. I had no idea
ich way was back to the camp site. I think I had walked at least 30 mins
d I wasn't even able to determine which direction I had come from. I was
ared, very scared to the point where I actually peed my pants. A nervousness
vel I had never felt before. It over came me and I was frozen and consumed
th fear. I panicked, started hyperventilating and shaking. I looked around
hopes of remembering my route, but nothing looked even remotely
miliar. At that moment, I noticed an extremely large Sequoia tree, 100 feet
vay. I decided that I was going to sit under that tree. It was the most
agnificent thing I had ever seen. I was this little object sitting under this
ant tree and that's when I told myself that I needed to get myself together

and figure out how to get back. I sat under that Tree for about 30 minut before I summoned up the courage to take action. I was now in a much calm state and I told myself that I could do this, that I could figure out with a cle mind how to navigate back. I had to believe in my instincts and I did. I look around and tried to rethink which direction I had come from. It was not a easy task when you have no markers or paths to follow. I don't really kno how I made it back, I think it was a mixture of my trust in my instincts an the fact that I was able to calm myself. When I got back, they had realiz that I was missing and were frantically looking around. I remember Mar commenting on how pale I looked. I usually look like I have a tan all ye long, but I was pale white from fear. Turned out, I was gone for over tw hours. I learned that day that I was capable of overcoming anything. I learn a huge lesson that day, to never underestimate what you are capable of doin I believed in my own capability and it got me out of what could have been disastrous situation, I could have gotten more lost, just by panicking.

Every day was like waking a dream. As a young child, I often da dreamed about the wilderness and how wonderful it would be to exist wi nature and here I am, living my dream. I went into my tent that night and was super charged from the day's events. My brain was racing with though of how fortunate and grateful I was to be able to get back to camp. It h happened where people get lost in these giant National Parks for weeks. I w unable to sleep that night, which was essential for a high-performan activity. Day four included a gain in elevation of 2400 feet.

Day Five was a vigorous day with a hike over the Muir Pass which h an elevation of 11,955 feet, with a rest at the top in a 75-year-old Stone H where there are signatures from hikers over many years, carved into the wal. After a brief rest, we started descending the Muir Pass which takes you in the Le Conte Canyon with huge vertical Granite Walls on either side. Th night at camp dinner, I had lost my appetite and had to force myself to e: Again, at sleep time, I was not able to sleep. The nights in your tent when y can't sleep are very long. I had run up the last portion of our way up the pa: as I wanted to test my endurance as it had greatly impacted my state of heal

Day Six, another grueling day with another hike over Mather Pass, a the toughest part of the hike so far 'The Golden Staircase,' which are swit

cks that are very steep and seemingly endless. They were exhausting to say
e least. Now I was starting to feel the effects of no sleep and very little food.
gain, at dinner time I had even less of an appetite, I ate very little and also
uld not sleep once again. My level of energy was declining quickly. I began
ignore what the inevitable reality was. I was getting very sick and in a grave
uation.

On Day 7, and after several nights of not sleeping and eating very little,
finally caught up to me. We had been hiking all morning and had finally
tten to a valley where we would have some lunch. I had absolutely no
petite what's so ever. I was not feeling very ill at this point. After sitting
ound for thirty minutes I got up to find a place to urinate. What I
perienced next was one of the most shocking moments I have ever had.
hen I looked down, I noticed that I was urinating pure blood. I was so
ared. I called Mark over because I couldn't believe what was happening.
y state of being was declining rapidly. I made the guides aware of what was
ing on and we decided that I should seek medical help. They arranged for
e to be taken out of the Mountains by Donkey the next day, which would
ve taken another day and a half to reach the exit of the park. My energy
rel was fading by the second but we had to move on. We started up hiking
ain and I was lagging behind at the back of the pack. I was struggling to the
int where I became delirious and was barely able to put one foot in front of
e other.

By this time, I had lost site of the group and I was in big trouble. The
xt thing I remember is waking up to a Paramedic kneeling over me. The
ides had access to a satellite phone and they were able to get a signal right
ay which is highly unusual, it could take many hours to get a signal. I had
llapsed on the trail and lost consciousness. The Paramedic was asking me
y name, I could hear what she was saying but I couldn't respond. I was put
to a stretcher and put into the helicopter. I'm now in the helicopter and I'm
lly aware of what's going on around me but unable to speak. The paramedic
d attached me to a heart monitor and I could hear my heart beat. It was
ating very fast and I also started to vomit violently. That's when the
ramedic radioed to her command that she thought I wasn't going to make
nd I needed to be transported to another helicopter that could get me to the
esno hospital in time in order to save my life. There happened to be a

helicopter available, sitting on the roof of Fresno hospital which was tl closest and best hospital for my particular condition. Another coincidence couldn't believe what I was hearing! I actually did not believe that I might, fact be dying. What! I was switched from the helicopter I was into a larg faster one and rushed to the roof of Fresno Hospital where I had my clothi cut off and tubes placed down my throat and the worst thing of all a cathete I was fighting to stay alive! I started to develop the worst head pain you cou imagine; it was like a regular head ache times a thousand. It felt like a ja hammer was drilling my head. Wow, it was intense. High Altitude Cerebr Edema, a swelling of the brain, was what was causing me such agony. At th point, I was high alert to everything going on around me. My senses had nev been so alive. Every sound was magnified, every visual was in slow motic and every second felt like a year. One of the fantastic doctors that were savi my life whispered in my ear when he must have seen me in such a high lev of pain He said and I quote "I know you can make it, I know how tough y are, you can make it through this, come on come on!" That was exactly wh he whispered in my ear and it's what has kept me alive. The next 24 hou were a complete blank to me. I regained conscience and I was lying on a b in a hospital room not really fully aware of where I was. I was on the highe amounts of Morphine possible and was in a state of hallucination. On t second day of being in the hospital in the afternoon I was taken for sever tests including an MRI to determine if there was any brain damage a CT sc to check my Kidneys and I was put into a Hydrostatic Water Tank th measures your body composition. It was determined that I did have swellii of the brain, however no brain damage and severe Dehydration that effect my kidneys. The reason I was urinating blood was because my kidneys we starting to fail. The other factor that was determined was that I had 5% bo fat, which in itself is very dangerous. My body fat was so low because pri to going into the mountains I already had very low body fat, in fact that is o of the reasons for my decline, not enough body fat for high altitude hiking.

On the third day, the Doctor came in the room and informed me on wh had happened. He basically told me that I was lucky to be alive and that the was nothing more the hospital could do and I needed weeks of rest. I discharged me with a page filled with instruction of what to do and what n to do. One of which was not to fly for at least two weeks, until the Bra swelling was completely normal. He also said that the only reason that I was able to survive my **near-death experience** was a direct result of me, being so physically fit. I survived the odds as a result of my **discipline** to my **health** and **well-being, period! All the physical and mental strength for which I worked so hard over the years, was finally paying off big time.**

I went back to the Motel where I had just arrived 7 days earlier. I was very slow and still very out of it. I could hardly gather my thoughts to check into the motel. I got to my room closed the door got into bed and slept for 10 hours. I awoke to the reality of what had just happened and it hit me like a brick wall. I was over whelmed with all sorts of emotions. I was angry and disappointed in myself. I then got up and went into the bathroom and saw myself for the first time. There were no mirrors in the Hospital bathrooms and I now realized why. I looked at myself in the mirror and I cried for two hours straight.

I looked like death. My face was all swollen from the drugs and my head was much larger than normal. I looked like a Freak Act in the Circus. At the same time the phone is now ringing constantly and the motel staff knocking on the door, making sure I was still alive. It turned out that my family was trying to call me and I wasn't picking up the phone so they got an employee of the Motel to bang on the door. I opened the door and assured him that I was alive. I just could not talk. After several hours of resting, I summoned up the energy to call my family. My wife had been informed by the travel company of my situation and was told that I was in critical condition. I spoke briefly to my Father and Sister and then I needed more sleep. This time I slept for 12 hours and I was starting to regain some energy. After three nights in the hotel, I wanted out. Marks friend Tim who drove us all to Fresno in Marks pickup truck was back in L.A. staying at Marks apartment. Tim is the son of the late Academy award winning Actress Susan Hayward. I contacted him and he drove out to get me in Fresno which is a 3 ½ hour drive. He took me back to the apartment in L.A., where I barely got out of my coach bed for 7 days. I had told my family not to come and see me. I didn't want any one around me I needed to recover. I was in a really bad place. My mind was filled with negative thoughts. I was in a very bad emotional state and I could not walk further than the bathroom and back to the bed, I didn't have the ability to do any of the everyday things we take for granted.

Luckily, I was being taken care of by Mark's neighbour and Tim, to whom I am forever grateful. They checked on me several times every day brought me food. On the third day of lying in bed in the apartment Tim came by to check on me. He thought it would be a good idea to get out to the local coffee shop, he could see that I was slipping into a deep dark place. According to Tim I was incoherent at the coffee shop not able to speak or move, it took me 15 mins to walk to the car from the coffee shop which was only 25 feet away. He was concerned and took me back to the apartment where he lay me on the couch. He waited with me until he was comfortable that I was going to be ok. A couple of days later I woke up starting to feel physically better but my mind was still in a bad place. I wasn't talking to any one, I had no motivation to do anything.

Later that day in the early evening there was a knock on the door. I was hesitant to answer at first, I was lying on the coach feeling sorry for myself but the knocking was persistent. Answering the door that night was one of the most important moments towards my recovery, it was the beginning. I wasn' eating very much and I looked emaciated. Two dear friends of mine had been informed of my condition and they came by to Take me back to their home in the Hollywood hills for a proper meal. They would not allow me to say no and I didn't resist. Wendel and her husband Patrick who knows a thing or two about cooking took me to their home and cooked me a wonderful meal. The best food I had had in a long while, I needed it. Wendel had been a dear friend of mine for forty years. She was always a great source of logic and truth, when I was in need of some advice. She approached issues with a certain calmness and rational that I always admired. She was a person that I truly authentically listened to, a very special person in my life. There was not a person in the World that was more suited to knocking on the door that evening than Wendel. She was the only person I would have listened to. Probably the only person that could talk some sense into me and she did just that. After dinner Wendel looked at me and I started crying. She let me cry for as long as needed. I think I cried for about 15 minutes. She then asked me in the softest most sympathetic tone "What are you thinking, what thoughts are in your head?" I told her that I felt like a loser and I let myself down, by not finishing the hike. I was still consumed with anger. She looked into my eyes and said "Are you kidding me, you just went on a much larger journey than climbing e mountain and finishing the trail, you just survived dying." A light went f in my head and that was the beginning of my mental recovery. Wendel is right, there was a much bigger picture to this experience and I was not eing it. I left Patrick and Wendell house a different person than when I went It was a very intimate and organic evening of healing for me. After dinner ey both took me back to the apartment where I had the best night sleep in eeks. I am forever grateful two both Wendel and Patrick.

Wendel passed away in January 2021. I will always hold within me, her ords of wisdom, her charm, creativity, passion and logic until the day I die. endel was a tremendously gifted actress with impeccable comedic timing. ie can be most remembered for her character of the low talker on the puffy irt episode of Seinfeld.

I progressively began to feel better. I started walking to the local coffee op although it took me three times longer than normal to get there. Over the an of forty-eight hours I was a different person. Ten days had gone by and w mark was coming to the end of his hike the summiting of Mt Whitney. m was scheduled to pick up Mark in a small California town called Lone ne. Lone Pine is where a great many old Hollywood Westerns were filmed. is located at the portal to Mt Whitney which is about 12 miles away. Mark d known idea as to what my outcome was. You can't communicate once u're deep on the trail. Tim asked me if I was up to going back to Lone Pine d surprising Mark. I jumped all over that opportunity. It is a 210-mile drive.

We departed in the Morning early, and had breakfast at a famous truck op in the middle of nowhere. It's where all the truckers eat. Great Food. ark and the rest of the hikers that were a part of my group was scheduled to ive in Lone Pine Early in the afternoon. Tim and I arrived around noon and ecked into the local Days Inn as we knew we were staying the night. A autiful full view of Mt Whitney with its magnificent jagged carved out ges was right behind the Motel. We walked the main street which is a etch of stores about 1/2 mile long and walked over to the motel were Mark, d all the others were booked into. They had already arrived and were in eir rooms. Funny coincidence Mark, was staying in the Susan Hayward om of the motel that had all of its rooms named after popular western actors io who had spent time in Long Pine. We knocked on the door Mark, was shocked

73

to see me alive. He thought there was a chance that I hadn't made it. It w
fantastic to be reunited with Mark and share our experiences with each othe
That night there was a dinner in Lone Pine to reunite with the rest of tl
hikers, which I attended. It was nice to see them again, they were all ve
curious about my journey. After dinner we were all very tired so we we
back to our motels and hit the sack as they say. We awoke early and Tim
Mark and I drove to that same truck stop and had the same amazing breakfa:
Then back to Marks apartment. I stayed in loss Angles with Mark for anoth
week in order to recover enough to fly home to Toronto. My condition w
improving every day. I was getting stronger, eating well and I was excited
return home to my Family.

After two weeks of recovery, I was ok to travel. So, after being aw:
from my family for three weeks I was on my way home. I arrived late th
night in Toronto and was greeted by my Wife and my Dog Terry who at th
time was only two and is now still alive at 161/2 years old. I am and was ve
appreciative of being able to get back Home. It took me a couple of mont
to get somewhat back to my previous self. After six months I was itching
have been physically and mentally challenged, so I started Boxing again
joined a Boxing Club and trained several hours a day. I Boxed for five yea
straight at a very high level. On my 50th birthday I was in Los Angel
Training with an ex-champion Boxer named Ricky Quills. He was a friei
and had been Trained by Freddie Roach, the greatest Boxing Trainer on Eart
Freddie trained Manny Pacquiao, Mike Tyson and many more great Boxei
Ricky arranged for me to go to Freddie's Gym wild card in North Hollywoc
It was amazing to have been trained for the day by Freddie and his Broth
Pepper and an ex-boxer named One Eye. He lost his eye in a fight. What
experience that was. I did a lot of sparing over the years and had one Amate
Fight. Which is exactly what I wanted to do. I was Fifty, but still as fit as ev
I made an agreement with my father-in-law Jim, who is now close to his 9!
Birthday, a man I love dearly. I was in my mid-twenties and we were standi
on the front porch of his Long Island New York Home. I was a big eater th
but I was also very active and working out so I never gained any weight. I
looked at me and said if I continue to eat that way that I will be a 220-pou
person, at the time I was 165 pounds and very lean. I told him that I will nev
gain weight in my life and that I will always maintain the same waist siz

n 60 years old now and I still have the same 30-inch waist I had in my mid-
enties. I also maintained the same weight 165 pounds my entire Life. Evert
ιe I see him I remind him of our bet.

Not until most recently, I started really thinking about what happened to
ε that day in the Mountains. More importantly how was I affected and what
d I learn. When I speak to people about that day most are very curious in
gard to what did I see (a white light). No lights, no gates. There is one aspect
out my experience that is most profound to me and that is, you're never
ore alive than when you're dying! All you want to have, is a good life. Life
about falling down, Living is getting back on your feet and standing up!!
ɔu never know how far you are from anything in life, opportunity and fate
ε waiting around every corner. An actors next audition might be his big
eak, a gold miners next swing of his axe might be his pot of gold. I could
ve **never believed that on the seventh day of our hike I would be in a**
ιlicopter fighting to stay alive.

"The Journey is not about the number of peaks you summit but abo every step you take to the summit," William Brian Sved

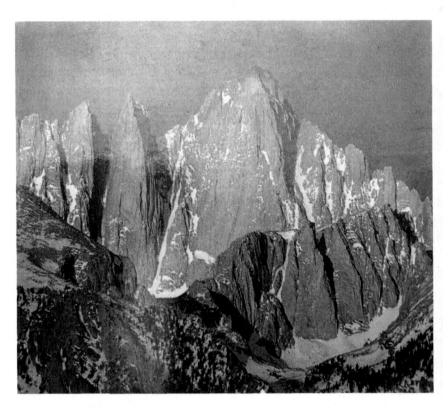

Mount Whitney, 14,505 feet

VII

BALANCE AND HARMONY

Balance, "Mental or Emotional stability. Harmony of Design and proportion. A situation in which different elements are equal or in the correct proportion."

Harmony, "Internal calm"

On one of my many visits to Joshua Tree National Park in southern California, very close to Palm Springs. Joshua Tree, is a magical place with magical energy. The silence of the desert always has a coming effect on my soul. On this particular visit my Son Montgomery, Mark and his son Luke embarked on a four-day adventure of hiking and climbing. We pitched our tents in one of the designated camping grounds within the Park. On the second day we hiked a 3-mile trail that Leeds to one of the highest points in the park called Ryan. Rather than take the trail we all chose the hardest route up, which was straight up the face of the mountain. It was one of the hardest things I have ever done. I had sprained my ankle earlier in the day and it swelled up like a grapefruit. That didn't stop me from keeping up. It took around an hour to reach the top. The view of the park from so high up is always the reward for a tough hike. Also at the top was a formation of rocks stacked one ontop of the other. There were small rocks with much larger rocks balanced on top. The entire formation of rocks was approximately six feet tall. It was amazing to see all these rocks perfectly balanced on top of one another. It was balance at perfection. There is a tremendous power of strength in perfect balance. When an athlete is well balanced in mind and body that athlete is so much more capable and has far less chance of injury.

I think to some extent life itself is about balance, nature certainly is. When a river is polluted the entire Ecosystem that is dependent on that source of water is affected. When a cars alignment is out of balance it will eventually have an effect on the entire car. The rubber tires will wear out quicker, the steering will be off. Balance applies to humans the same way it does to the car and the river. Everything works in harmony when it is balanced.

Street performers use balance in their acts. Riding a unicycle or juggling pins require practice. The more you practice the more capable you become. The same theory can be said for balance. Most people live in some regard an unbalanced lifestyle, too much of one thing and not enough of another. It is important to be able to identify where your lifestyle might be out of balance and that's difficult. In my many years of Training most of my clients were not able to identify their in-balances.

Do you sleep too much or too little, eat too much, and drink too little water, sit too long and stand too little, work too much and socialize too little and the list goes on. The most important balance is between the Body and the Mind.

One of the reasons that I relished the opportunity to hike and climb to high altitudes in the middle of nowhere was because I developed a ritual. Where ever Mark and I hiked we would find either a bolder or mountain of some sort to climb up. When you get to the top of a high peak it's like you have a window looking into the amazing thing that nature is. It really puts things in perspective. It allows you the opportunity to realize how small and insignificant we really are. I developed a ritual that I would stand at the top of whatever peek we had climbed and I pretended that I was throwing away all my mental garbage all the nonsense I was holding onto. I actually performed a mimic as if I was really throwing a bag of garbage away. It was very helpful for me. When I returned to life in the big city after being in the desert, it always allowed me to put things in perspective. It balanced me. Gave me a sense of harmony.

If you spend the majority of your time in a high stress, high energy state mentally, it will ultimately lead to physical issues. There has to be a balance. Many years ago, I was training an emergency room nurse. Really sweet man. He was a very eager client and had tremendous results from training together. After about a year he suggested that we develop an exercise and stretch class for other nurses in the hospital. It was a good idea so I pursued it. I met with the head of the dept and they thought it a good idea as well. They gave me a room in the basement I posted a notice on the bulletin board and before I knew, I had twenty nurses signed up. Being an emergency nurse is a super high stress environment. The class which was 40 minutes gave them all a sense of balance that allowed them more tolerance to their job.

Having a more balanced lifestyle will reward you. There is a strength in balance and a very certain harmony. It' actually a very powerful aspect of anything. Without balance you would not be able to walk. It has a very positive effect on your well-being.

How aware are you? Do you pay attention to your environment? How aware are you of yourself? I am a self-admitted absolute Marlon Brando, The Godfather freak. He is the reason I pursued a career as an actor. Brando was one of the most aware humans to date. What made him such a talented actor was his ultra-awareness of himself and also his environment. After his death in 2004, Sean Penn was interviewed the day after his death, he was a close friend. He gave a great eulogy and told a story about if Brando was in a room with ten flies buzzing around, he would know where all ten flies where and what they were doing while he was talking to you. I have encountered moments in my life where I was so focused and aware of myself and my environment, it was like life was moving in slow motion and I was in total control of all the energy around me. On one such occasion I was doing a scene in my favorite acting teachers class, her name was Elaine Aiken. Elaine was a teacher at Lee Strasberg School. After a couple of months of studying with her she decided to leave the school and create her own class, with the help of the late great actress Shelly Winters, which was in Hell's Kitchen. It was one the worst neighbourhoods in Manhattan. The class ended late most nights and I would run a couple of avenues just to get to a street that had working lights. She was the sweatiest most companionate person. I really enjoyed performing for her. I was doing a scene from a play called 'Street Car Named Desire.' It was a very aggressive scene it does get physical. However, as an actor it's important to realize your boundaries. That night I experienced the most connected I had ever been as an actor. It's like you're pushing yourself through a vortex and stripping down all the things that hold you back. Its complete freedom. I was so focused and aware of everything, I was hyper aware, I am a hyper aware junky! Ultra focus has always intrigued me. I remember watching a street performer play the harmonica in NYC, he was so focused on his instrument that life around him didn't exist. I will always remember the way that he played that harmonica, the focus he had.

I had an actor friend in NYC, his name was Roberto. Roberto, was the most screwed up guy around. His personal life was a mess. He had no mother and a Father who was super abusive. I remember he showed up at school one day after being on a binge for several weeks, he looked like a complete mess. He was however the most talented human being I have ever known. He was an actor on the level of a Brando. This guy was one cool dude. He could play any instrument and sing and dance like a rock star. One day he and I were walking down 5th Ave near Washington Square Park, it was fall and a little bit cold so he was wearing a very tattered coat (he never had any money, that had chalk stains all over.) We stopped in front of a big old apartment building and he turns and looks at me and points to a place for me to sit and says, "I'm going to paint something on the sidewalk, just hang out and watch." He kneels on the ground and pulls out a bunch of chalk from either of his stained pockets and starts creating a Frame for his drawing. He also puts his hat, which was also stained from chalk on the ground in front of him and starts working on his art. I sat there in complete amazement as Roberto drew from memory a perfect Mona Lisa. Pedestrians looked at him drawing in complete wonderment when they realized he was creating from memory. I sat there watching the reactions of people. It was incredible. The entire time that he was creating he did not look up from his concrete canvas once. He too was ultra focused and aware, there wasn't a moment wasted in this guy's life. He lived every moment to its fullest When we left his hat was filled with money, probably a hundred bucks Being a student of acting gave me an opportunity to explore my emotions and dig deep into self-awareness. Being a thespian in and of itself is the ability to be as real and alive as possible in a moment. One of the most challenging aspects of life is to live in every moment, not live in the past or future.

How aware are you?

1. What are your triggers? What strategies do you use to calm yourself?

2. What are the things about yourself you enjoy and what are the things you don't enjoy.

3. What really stresses you. What are your inner core beliefs?

4. When you are out in nature how aware are you of your space. Do you see the sky and trees. People today face a tremendous number of challenges on a daily basis. Their problems don't become smaller ,their stress levels don't change, but if your mind and body are stronger problems and stress levels are a lot more manageable. To learn more about yourself and develop the ability to control and regulate your emotions and to understand your inner truth will give you Peace of mind.

Self-Care

Physical:

1. Sleep.

2. Stretching.

3. Walking.

4. Exercise.

5. Healthy food choices.

6. Rest.

Emotional:

1. Manage Stress.

2. Forgiveness.

3. Positive thinking.

4. Compassion and Kindness.

Social:

1. Set boundaries.

2. Positive support from others.

3. Communication.

4. Social Interaction.

Spiritual:

1. Time alone.

2. Connection with nature.

3. Expressing your thoughts.

4. Being more aware of your environment.

When I was studying acting at The Lee Strasberg school, one of our teachers gave us a challenge. The challenge was that you could not shower for a week, could not brush your teeth or wash your face or change your cloths. Well let me tell you something, when you smell and look dirty people begin to treat you completely different. That was what the exercise was about. You become tremendously aware of yourself and how people view you.

An old friend of mine, Duke Redbird an Ojibwa, an indigenous elder wise man, and author once told me, "You have to want what you get and not always get what you want." It always stuck with me. It made sense to me. You should always appreciate the things you have. If you don't appreciate what you have, it will never matter how many things you acquire.

What you think, you become.

What you feel, you attract.

What you imagine, you create.

- BUDDA

Five years ago, I was parked on a main street in the city waiting in my car while the car in front of me finished parallel parking her car. She was a young college student that was driving her sisters brand new Jeep. She backed right into the front of my car gave it a real good smack. We both got out and there was a lot of damage to my car and not a scratch to hers. She was very nervous and started crying, so I calmed her down and assured her not to worry. She had no money and it wasn't even her own car. I thought about it for a moment and decided to give her a break. I told her to just forget about the damages to my car and that I would take care of it. I didn't really like my car at the time and I really didn't care about how it looked. The front bumper was hanging off. It was more important to me to be kind to this young girl who was in a panic. The only thing I asked of her was that she promise me that she will pass on the favor to someone else one day. She promised that she would and I drove away. When I got home, I ducked taped the bumper back on the car and left it that way until I finally sold the old clunker. Every time I looked at that bumper it reminded me of my good deed.it made me feel grounded. The energy that you put out is the energy you will receive back.

In 1983, when I lived in Los Angeles. My wife used to work in Beverly Hills and I would often drive her to work on my way to school. I would normally grab a coffee and a bagel from my favorite spot, Bagel Nosh on little Santa Monica Blvd. There was a homeless man, living behind the shop. Every morning I also bought him a bagel and coffee. I didn't have a lot of money at that time but non the less doing that gave me a sense of well-being. One day after about a year of supplying his morning breakfast he came up to me and asked if tomorrow we could go to the Mexican restaurant down the street. There was a Mexican restaurant in Beverly Hills called the Red Onion and it was high end Mexican food that I could not afford for even myself. Not long after that he disappeared. Participating in the betterment of yourself and other living creatures' manifests into positive energy. Random acts of kindness create a feeling of honor and well-being!

When Whitman wrote, "I sing the body electric"

I know what he meant,

I know what he wanted,

To be completely alive every moment,

In spite of the inevitable.

We can't cheat death but we can make it work so hard

that when it does take us,

It will have known a victory,

just as perfect as ours.

Charles Bukowski,

1920-1994

85

Checkout our merchandise at http://www.muscle-head.com

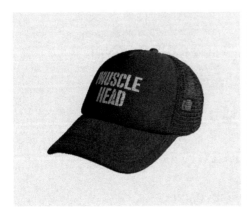

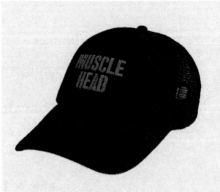

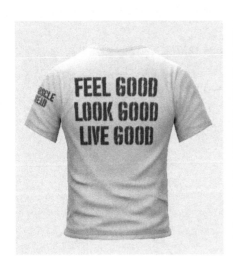

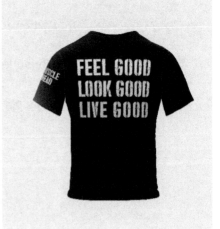

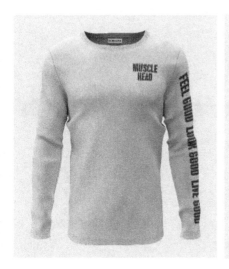
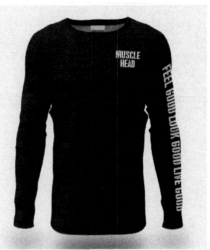
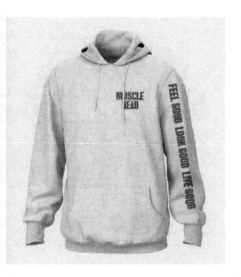
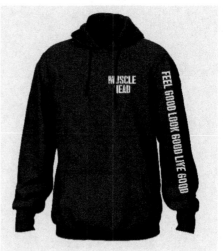

87

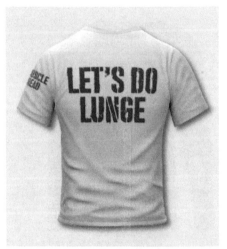

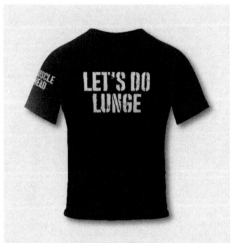

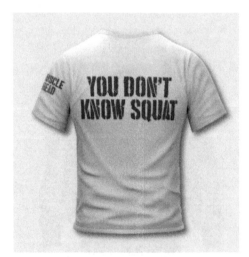

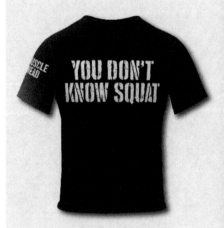

88

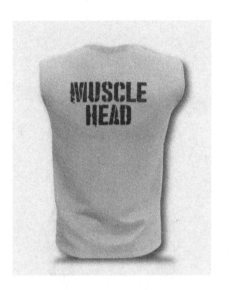

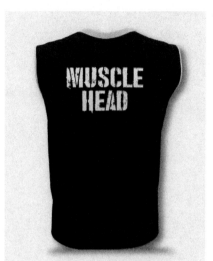

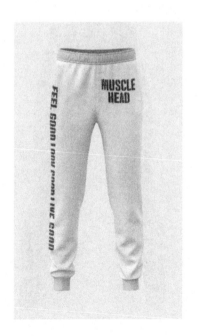

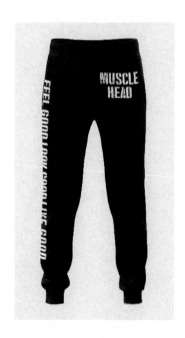

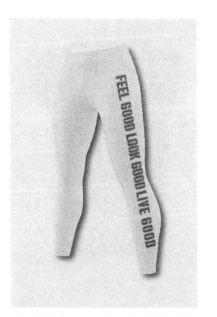

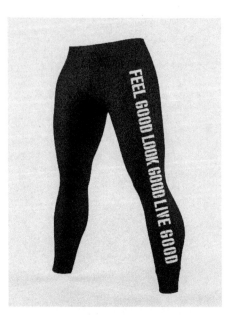

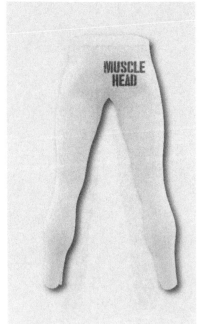

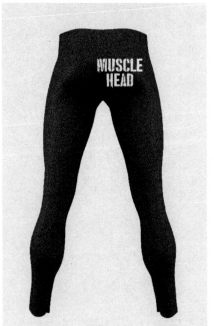

Printed in Great Britain
by Amazon

34905087R00056